Faith, Hope, & Cancer

A Survivor's Tips

Carol Westfahl

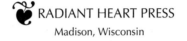

RADIANT HEART PRESS
Madison, Wisconsin

Copyright © 2006 by Carol Westfahl.
All rights reserved.

Published by:
Radiant Heart Press
(an imprint of Goblin Fern Press, Inc.)
6401 Odana Road, Suite B
Madison, WI 53719
Toll-free: 888-670-BOOK (2665)
www.goblinfernpress.com

ISBN-10: 1-59598-037-7
ISBN-13: 978-1-59598-037-3
Library of Congress Cataloging Number:
2006932173

Library of Congress Cataloging-in-Publication
Data available on request.

Cover art by Jessica Lehry Miller

Typography and book design by Sential Design,
www.sentialdesign.com

Printed in the United States of America.

*For Joyce,
my friend and editor*

Contents

Foreword i
Preface iii
Introduction v
Timeline vii

I. Heaven Help Me 1

    1. My Wake-Up Call 3
    2. The Diagnostic Process 11
    3. Choices in Treatment 21
    4. Chemo—Strong Medicine 29

II. We Can Cope 37

    5. Fight for Life 39
    6. No Passive Victims 47
    7. Does Anyone Care? 57
    8. Prayer and People 71

III. I Will Survive 77

    9. Build on Success 79
    10. Ask the Experts 85
    11. Options in Therapy 93
    12. Dealing With Stress 109
    13. Focus on Others 115

IV. To Heal Again 119

  14. Mom, My Hero... 121
  15. Power of Faith 127
  16. I'm Still Me.. 137
  17. Gift from God 143

Acknowledgements 149

A Survivor's Tips

  1. Coping Skills for the Patient 19
  2. Cancer Truisms 27
  3. How Can You Help?.................................. 64
  4. Know Before You Go................................. 67
  5. What Not to Say to the Patient.................. 68
  6. My Resources for Getting Well 75
  7. Immune System Boosters......................... 112
  8. What Cancer Taught Me.......................... 141

And life is what we make it,
always has been, always will be.
—Grandma Moses

Foreword

Carol is a true survivor and has beaten cancer as far as I am concerned, and beating it is not about curing it or becoming immortal. It is about not becoming a victim. Carol instinctively, and with coaching, did the right things; including wanting to throw my book away while reading a question I asked, "What are the benefits of having this disease?" That is survival behavior, and that anger is energy, and energy can be used to heal whereas depression and fear accomplish nothing except self-destruction.

Carol has learned, and her book relates, the importance of the combination of inspiration and information, and that is what survivors do. Carol is a native who can share the experience that tourists, who have not been in cancerland, cannot understand. She knew that coaching helps performers but they, like you, have got to be willing to put in the time to achieve their goals and become stars. For me, the survivor will exceed expectations because of the life they are living, which comes with an acceptance of one's mortality—like quitting a job as she did when learning of a recurrence of cancer.

Some people see their parents, teachers, and God as punishing, creating guilt, shame and blame. Carol saw beyond that. I hope those readers who did not feel love as a child will re-parent themselves and realize God does not create afflictions. Cancer is a loss of health. God, family, and health-care professionals all are trying to help you find your health again.

So read what Carol has to say and use her as a role model for change and healing. She has created a guidebook for cancer patients.

—Bernie S. Siegel, M.D.

Preface

Faith, Hope and Cancer: A Survivor's Tips is an extraordinarily good book that integrates one woman's reflections on cancer recovery.

Carol Westfahl was the architect of her own healing. In this eloquent treatment memoir, she takes us from the ground floor, "You have cancer," to the penthouse of her multi-faceted, hands-on healing process. Whether you have cancer or know someone who does, Carol's story will enlighten and inspire you.

Like a phoenix rising after her initial diagnosis, Carol conquered her cancer and achieved remission, only to have it recur years later. Her gutsy, yet poignant account of her return to health is remarkable and uplifting. With determination and a supportive treatment team, Carol courageously reminds us that life often means change. Cancer can be a powerful precursor to awaken your positive spirit within. She guides us through her own personal growth and gives many resources to help cancer patients create their own blueprint for healing.

—Judith B. Krings, Ph.D.

Introduction

The real story in this book is not just about my battles with cancer, but about you, the reader, and how you will respond to crisis in any form—yours or that of one you love. All of us want to respond compassionately to those desperately in need of tender, loving care. During a health crisis the importance of our relationships cannot be over-emphasized. Family and friends become even more important as our support team.

What do we say and do when others are looking to us for wisdom, guidance, and answers? Words likely do not come easily, seem inadequate, or at times remain unsaid. There are many ways to relate to people who find themselves in circumstances they didn't plan, but now hope to survive. We just aren't sure how to relate. There is no formula for doing it right. We can learn to reach out to others at critical times in their lives.

It's possible to survive adversity of any type and do it with dignity. We can remain true to ourselves by taking responsibility for decisions affecting our health and well-being. I am living proof that this is possible. I write out of respect for the ill, who more than anything, want to regain normalcy.

This is my account of living with a life-threatening disease. But it's more than telling my story. It's a book of ideas I tested personally to ease distress as I searched for answers. I also share practical suggestions that may make it easier for you to talk with those experiencing a health crisis.

My story is interspersed with the lessons I learned. They are included, as it is impossible to gloss over the complex emotional and physical issues faced by patients. Recurring themes are communication and the loving support of family and friends. I believe a combination of efforts helped me beat cancer into remission, and this book focuses on those topics.

Section One speaks of facing the news of a life-threatening illness. Chapters in Section Two speak to those newly-diagnosed and their needs. It explores basic concepts of interpersonal communication. The third section details options in therapy, in addition to traditional treatments. It suggests learning from the experts who influenced my thinking and recovery. The final section covers the spiritual aspect of our miraculous lives.

My strong faith in God was a significant factor in my struggle with cancer, so I have included

INTRODUCTION

appropriate Bible verses that comforted me. May these verses touch you in a way that eases your journey.

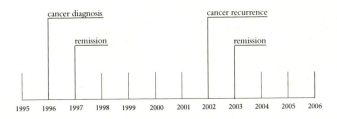

My Journey of Faith and Hope

~I~

Heaven Help Me

*Nothing in all creation is
hidden from God's sight.*

—Hebrews 4:13

~1~

My Wake-Up Call

The day I received the news I had cancer was literally the "first day of the rest of my life." Life as I knew it was gone, forever changed. Cancer caught up to me, as it did my parents. Was it inevitable? Was it in the genes? In my heart I always feared it could come to this. The forty-five days it took to diagnose seemed endless. Tests. Waiting. More tests. More waiting.

I received word via telephone while at work. The innocent question, "Are you sitting down?" spoke volumes. I sat down. I held my breath. My physician very calmly detailed what I was facing. When she finished speaking my life was askew, on tilt. I was in an unknown world. My mind was racing. I didn't cry. I've no idea how I made it through the rest of that day.

What a jolt it was! I thought I was going to die. How much time did I have? My father only had two weeks between diagnosis and his death from acute leukemia. I didn't sleep those first two weeks as I struggled to put my life in order, just in case that was all the time I had. If I did doze off, the minute I opened my eyes I started crying. It was automatic, and there was no holding back. I was feeling very sorry for myself. My feelings of isolation were overwhelming. Who could I trust with this information? Who could possibly understand what I was going through? Where did I go from here? What next?

A diagnosis of stage IV non-Hodgkins lymphoma was reached early in February of 1996. Lymphoma is a disease of the immune system, or more accurately, a weakened immune system. The bad news about lymphoma is that there is no cure. The good news is that it is supposedly one of the easiest to put into remission. Easy? I don't think so! There is nothing easy about treatment.

Chemotherapy is difficult and damaging, to say the least. The oncologist insisted we begin treatment in early March. I had asked if we could delay treatment. He said, "No." My son was getting married that month and I was concerned about hair loss. Vanity! My hair started falling a few days before the wedding. I woke up numerous

My Wake-Up Call

times during the night, checking to see if my hair was on the pillow or on my head.

It was a long, agonizing journey for me from the initial devastation of diagnosis in February to the miraculous news of remission at the end of 1996. As a follow-up, I submitted to routine testing for six years. Initially it was every six months. As time went on, testing was reduced to once a year. I never was able to block out the entire experience, but I did start to trust my body again.

Then in September of 2002, another devastating blow—the monster was back. Routine testing showed a recurrence of lymphoma. That famous "five-years and cured" standard may apply to certain types of cancer, but not to lymphoma. It was just as shocking to hear the news the second time. I was totally unprepared for it. I was speechless. Air left the room. I felt as if I were suffocating. I couldn't get out of that building fast enough. My first impulse was actually just to run...pack my car and leave...maybe drive to Arizona and live in the desert on berries and nuts. I was frantic and stunned beyond belief. My mind was screaming, *No, it can't be true. I cannot go through this again!! I can't!! I will not do it!*

In my darkest moments I simply could not fathom subjecting myself to treatments a second time. But, of course, I did. It took even more courage the second go around because I already knew the drill. So it started over—the PET scan; endless blood tests; the infinite appointments. Negative images flooded my mind. I remembered the final treatment in 1996 when a vein being used for chemo collapsed half-way through. My veins had been ravaged. There was no way they could be used again. How could I survive this? A PICC line was said to be the answer. However, the attempt to install the line failed after four agonizing hours. The line could not be threaded past my collarbone, which I had broken in a fall as a child.

    The clock was ticking again. I had been scheduled to begin chemo when the PICC line failed. I agonized over the decision to start chemo treatment prior to having a port installed because I knew it would be difficult to find a vein to carry the chemo. What to do? This time my oncologist left the decision to me whether to delay treatment or attempt to find a vein. I hoped to rid myself of this new monster as quickly as possible. So, after careful consideration, I was scared but I showed up for the appointment. A very competent nurse brought my veins to the surface. She took her time and selected a vein that worked. Her patience and helpfulness gave me courage. Watching her calm demeanor reinforced my belief in good people and my good fortune to work with experts.

My Wake-Up Call

It doubled my determination to fight as hard as the first time.

As we waited for my white counts to climb following that treatment, a port was scheduled to be installed into my chest. A port is a device that is used to administer chemo and to draw blood. My right lung was punctured during this procedure. There was a one percent chance that could happen, and it did. The pain was excruciating. I did appreciate my oncologist's great sense of humor when he told me chemo would be a breeze compared to that experience. None of this was funny, but we both laughed. Sometimes black humor is better than no humor at all.

I saw the first diagnosis as a warning. I needed to slow down and change my priorities. The second diagnosis was a God moment. This is it! This time I realized I had no time to waste. I responded instantly, "Okay God. I get it. I finally get it." I believed that He was in charge of my life and would be handling all my problems. I suddenly knew He would be with me all the way.

This personal wake-up call from God was the greatest learning experience of my life. This period was a time of quiet growth for me. It was a period of solitary reading and research. I spent much time alone, especially following treatment. I retired from my job within weeks of the second diagnosis. Retirement gave me the time I needed to examine my life, to direct my limited energy towards health, towards getting my life in order, and towards preparing for whatever the future held. Both the first and second diagnosis brought forth questions about the end of life. I recall a quiet conversation with my children in which I told them never to feel bad for me because I'd had a wonderful life.

I cannot say that cancer was a totally negative experience. It served as a teacher and I was its student not once, but twice. I was, however, haunted by a need to discover what lessons I missed the first time that sent me back to square one. There are no answers to that riddle. I had to get past it and move on. There simply was nothing more I could have done to prevent a recurrence. I had taken recovery very seriously and worked hard to regain my former strength and stamina. In my six years of remission I'd been totally aware that each day was a gift from God. The message I offered to those looking for answers was that cancer is not a death sentence. I was a living example that survival was possible.

Cancer changed my mindset and my perception of life itself. Cancer made me question what life is about. It asked me: "What is really important? Why are you here? What is the meaning of life? What

My Wake-Up Call

is your mission?" It invited me to contemplate my life—both the past and present, and my possible future. It stunned me into silence and forced me to listen for the quiet inside.

The wake-up call pushed me to the edge where only the important things come into focus. Material things didn't and don't seem to matter as much. I had to believe things happened for a reason. Life is brief; time is of the essence and cannot be wasted. I developed an acute awareness of living in the moment. My choices were to grumble about my health or rejoice I was alive. I want to live life without regrets. I no longer engage in long-range planning or take anything for granted. I savor my memories.

I learned to control what I could, but the truth is that I controlled very little. The knowledge that cancer could occur again makes my future uncertain—just like everyone else's. I found that by turning my problems over to the Lord, I no longer needed to fret over them. I'm convinced it's all taken care of for me.

*For we are his workmanship,
created in Christ Jesus
for good works, which God prepared beforehand
that we should walk in them.*
—Ephesians 2:10

~2~

The Diagnostic Process

Health is our wealth. Serious illness rocked my very foundation. With cancer, I felt betrayed by my own cells. I was left alone, face-to-face with reality. Every cancer experience is unique. Only I could decide the right course of treatment for my cancer. In the final analysis, it was my project, but I needed lots of love and support. I had to trust in my ability to reason and trust the Wisdom that created me. I needed to be willing to assume a proper share of responsibility for my own health and recovery; to be a partner and active agent in the treatment. My physical well-being was my constant concern.

In looking back at my life, I had thought of myself as a healthy person whose life was basically in order. I had three grown, productive children and five wonderful grandchildren. Life was good. I had a great job. I was into exercise and nutrition, eating steamed vegetables and plenty of fruit. I considered myself an optimist/realist, not a Pollyanna, but someone who saw the glass as half-full. Life was always on the upswing. Nothing about my health had suggested what lay ahead of me.

Then in 1995, wham! As I did floor exercises one morning, I discovered a mass tucked beneath the bottom of my rib cage. Imagine my horror! My day had been normal until that moment—then I reluctantly carried a gigantic question mark in my side. Its presence was impossible to ignore. I could think of nothing else. There was no separating *mass* and *cancer* in my mind. My mind was racing and it stopped me in my tracks. My family history had always made me cognizant of an increased risk. I remembered the devastation of treatment routines, having observed them firsthand with my mom. Now I was frightened! I knew life came with no guarantees. But it wasn't death I feared—it was the process of getting to that point. Thoughts of my parents' untimely deaths were in the front of my mind. How I wished I could talk to them.

I had to decide what to do about the mass. The timing for this discovery was so bad. Then again,

The Diagnostic Process

could there ever be a good time? It was December, and I was already running as fast as I could. The snowstorms were unrelenting; the weather was cold and cruel. The holidays were upon us. I needed time, but did I have it? Research was the answer, but when to do it? I was in a panic. I talked to myself constantly, "You will be rational, and you will be calm."

In the meantime, I was profoundly exhausted. I had no idea this was a symptom of lymphoma. I managed to get through the holidays without a peep to anyone and then began my research to identify the mass. Based solely on its location, my uneducated hypothesis was that it was a spleen problem. I called the clinic, explaining that I had a suspicious lump. Luckily an appointment was scheduled the very next day; unbeknownst to me, so was a spectacular ice storm. I was on the interstate highway for more than two hours, slip-sliding down the road, trying to keep the car on the icy pavement as I drove to the clinic.

I talked myself through the trip by saying, "Piece of cake; piece of cake; piece of cake compared to having cancer." What else could it be? The odds were not in my favor. When I finally arrived, the receptionist informed me I had missed my appointment. She offered me no options. I was desperate to see my doctor; it must have shown on my face as I explained the ice storm to those in the cocoon of the clinic. I was sure my doctor would see me if they would only ask her. I made the request and she did see me.

Following her examination I heard the chilling phrase, "We'll just run a few tests." A battery of blood tests was ordered. The empty halls in the clinic reflected the nasty weather outside. I sat alone as the seriousness of my situation sank in. I thanked God for my very competent doctor. She was concerned, even courteous enough to show interest in my spleen theory. That ray of hope kept me going for days. She also freely dispensed hugs—the best medicine.

Not wasting any time, a CT scan was scheduled within days at the tiny local hospital. The technician was professional, explaining the entire procedure, starting an IV, and then retreating into a glass room. I was left alone with the huge, sterile machine. I lay on the table as a recorded voice told me, "Take a deep breath and hold," or "You may breathe," as a laser beam rushed around me and the table inched forward into the machine. About halfway through the exam, the machine stopped and the tech entered the room with a question. "Were you ever in a car accident, or did you have surgery as a child?" He went on to explain there were differences in the bone mass on the left and right sides of my body. His question surprised me, but then I answered, "Oh yes—I had polio when I was two years old." He noted it for the radiologist who would read the films.

Within days the scan was followed by an ultrasound-guided needle biopsy at the local hospital. The room was jammed with curious medical types, none of whom introduced themselves to me. The attention this one little tumor was attracting made my imagination run wild. The ultrasound revealed a tumor the size of a grapefruit in my chest cavity tucked under the bottom of my rib cage. I asked to see it. There it was in living color on the screen. Now I knew the enemy! One look at the screen defined the tumor for me. That vision has stayed with me. It helped me gauge its size as treatment progressed. The biopsy was sent to the doctors at Mayo Clinic. After their analysis, I was instructed to hand-carry test results of all my preliminary tests to a large teaching hospital three hours away for the actual diagnosis.

My oldest son flew in to take me to my first appointment at the teaching hospital. We checked out this vast facility. The only remotely pleasant moment of the entire afternoon occurred at the admitting desk when the clerk asked if I had ever been a patient there. Their records revealed that I had been treated for polio in 1940. My confidence soared. However, good record-keeping does not equal excellence in patient care. That confidence plummeted when a nurse led me to a huge scale just off the waiting room. My weight and height were yelled out to anyone interested. It was tempting to ask if she would like to announce my shoe size or perhaps my bra size, as well. Later, on the trip home, my son said, "Well, now I know how much you weigh." We both had a good laugh about that.

During each of my two visits to that hospital I was examined by three doctors. I was asked if I objected to interns being present during the examinations, which I didn't. The interns were skeptical about my finding the mass myself. I attempted to be cooperative while responding to rapid-fire questions put forth by this medical entourage. My assigned doctor struck me as particularly ghoulish when she was absolutely delighted to announce the availability of an open bed in the chemo room to conduct a bone marrow test.

For that test, I was led into a large room which accommodated up to thirty people in various stages of treatment. I was horrified! I was led to an empty bed. I asked for the restroom, which is where I talked myself into staying and allowing

The Diagnostic Process

the procedure, knowing delay was not in my best interest. When I returned to the bed, I stated I was very uncomfortable with the lack of privacy. That said, the nurse offered to pull the curtain, which helped me immensely. Please, spare me just a little dignity.

Between visits to that hospital and after my assembly-line tests in those early days following the collapse of my world, all I wanted was silence so I could hear my own thoughts. I attempted to make sense of all the medical literature I was scanning. I struggled with the technical information provided by the teaching hospital. The printed information available on the chemotherapy drugs was so daunting and the side effects were so frightening. There was no time for explanations, just, "You need to read this." Treatment options required tremendous decision-making. I had neither the knowledge nor training to make informed choices. I was still dealing with my life coming apart at the seams.

My younger son took me to the hospital for the second visit. The doctors filed in and ticked off numbers, which meant nothing to me. They attached unfamiliar medical terms to the numbers. English, please! They were speaking another language. I had to ask questions about what I would want the numbers to be. It was nightmarish, but I wasn't dreaming. Their brief speech was clinical, detached, and delivered with less empathy than the artificial voice of the CT scanner. My questions were answered in likelihoods, probabilities, and statistics. I understood I was no longer a human being. I was whatever the diagnosis would show me to be.

I did doubt I had what it would take to survive. Through my reading I later learned that statistics are just numbers, numbers that reflect a range of possibilities. My questions centered on what I could do to survive this and get past it. I wanted to know what would make things better right now; what could I change? With my medical history, cancer was a probability I had lived with nearly all my life.

My primary care physician called after my first appointment at the diagnostic hospital. What a godsend she was to me! I told her it would be difficult for me to get well there. She patiently explained, "All we need from them is the diagnosis, and we can take it from there." I would return to her for medical treatment, her warm hugs, and advice.

Finally, after six weeks, lymphoma was confirmed. I knew the enemy. I then had frank discussions with my children, using the words *cancer* and *death*. That is when I started living with cancer, when I started developing my own coping skills.

Coping Skills for the Patient

1. Give yourself credit for surviving the diagnosis.
2. Attitude is everything. Fight for your life.
3. Maintain the interests important to you.
4. Do your own research.
5. Join a support group.
6. Be gentle with yourself.
7. Bring a friend or book with you to the clinic.
8. Record your conversations with your doctor.
9. Accept what the day brings.
10. Find a competent counselor.

The Lord has said, 'Never will I leave you;
Never will I forsake you.
—Hebrews 13:5

~3~

Choices in Treatment

I have always appreciated the positive manner in which my oncologist offers new products. Once past the initial shocking news of cancer, the person who most influenced the quality of my life was my oncologist. Over the course of my illness, my emotional and personal well-being was affected by the conversations I had with him. My level of stress decreased because I trusted, respected, and felt comfortable with him.

I believe when it comes to health decisions, the physician owes us a realistic assessment of the potential negative effects of treatment, be it surgery, chemotherapy, or radiation therapy. Care cannot be provided in the absence of reasonable explanations about health concerns, needs, finances, risks, and alternative options. Decisions about treatment require answers. As patients, we have the right to choose our treatment.

Basic questions to ask include:

1) What are the treatment goals?
Are there reasonable chemotherapy treatments for my cancer?

2) What is the treatment process?
Do these anti-cancer drugs have side effects?

3) What are the risks and benefits?
What is a realistic assessment of my future quality of life?

These questions may sound simplistic, but once addressed, I was in a better position to make reasonable choices about how to proceed. Not that I had a good understanding, but my physician gave me hope, thus making decisions easier. I think doctors need to explain all available options. As patients, we need understandable explanations of what is wrong with us and what can be done about it. I always asked for clarification when my doctor used terms or phrases I was not familiar with. I took notes. I had to write down the main points or I would have lost a huge percentage of what the doctor said. Good physicians listen, empathize, and hopefully understand that no one wants to be a patient. Warmth, understanding, and technical skills are the right combination in a doctor for me.

Adequate communication between the doctor and the patient is an essential part of healing. I wanted a physician with clinical ability; who was direct, yet reassuring about my situation; one who was committed to quality of life rather than quantity of life. I voiced my concerns, described symptoms I believed were important, and required explanations. I had to do my homework on procedures that were recommended. Surgery was not an option in my case because lymphoma affects systems throughout the body. I learned to be bold; my health is the most important thing I have. Which treatment goal is right for me? In the final analysis, a decision based on rational and accurate appraisals of the disease and prognosis lies with the patient—the right to informed consent.

We also have the right to die. Some doctors view death as an evil adversary and will attempt to sustain life at a high emotional cost to the patient. In many cases, people would opt for a humane approach that means a shorter life with relative comfort—choosing the right to die.

I was totally demoralized and without hope as I returned from the teaching hospital. My physician helped me make the decision to receive treatment locally. A supportive friend of mine attended my first appointment with the local oncologist. She provided for me a second set of ears, and her memory of details discussed was much better than mine. I will always be grateful for her help, and I strongly recommend taking someone along when meeting with a doctor.

I was impressed with the oncologist. He had an excellent reputation as a diagnostician and strong patient advocate. I liked his positive attitude. He assured me there were many options and we would find the right combination to combat this disease. He discussed the protocol and the reasons for the choice of drugs. His manner was calm, causing me to feel as comfortable as one could in those circumstances. I left that meeting with hope for the first time in months. I was blessed to have two very humane doctors looking after me. I rate both as "genius" on the skill/talent scale. They handled every problem I encountered with great skill, care, and compassion.

I lived with the uncertainty of my decisions, but I was not giving up—stage IV or not. Statistics do not penetrate the heart. I really wanted to be well. "Just do it," borrowed from Nike, became my motto. I never considered "do nothing" as an option. I had to give it my all. I wasn't denying the diagnosis, but I did think the jury was still out. All I could do was survive one day at a time and await the treatment outcome.

At first my illness affected everything. It took so much energy to be happy, sad, grateful, or horrified. Some days it was all just beyond me. The effects of the treatment were cumulative, so things continually deteriorated. I was dealing with so much while attempting to be positive about my future. I went through all the stages connected to illness and death. First is the denial, along with shock and numbness; the second stage is anger; third is bargaining; fourth is depression; and finally comes acceptance. Yes, I was angry. This is what I learned from it: directed anger can be empowering and invaluable for improving state of mind and health in general.

I recognized a strong correlation between my physical and mental state. I knew after reading the drug descriptions and side effects that I needed to change my mindset regarding the dangerous drugs used in chemotherapy. They are so very toxic. Fear of chemotherapy drugs is understandable because their toxic impact spills over onto healthy cells. I needed to reframe my view from that of *dangerous drug* to *drug of choice* if I wanted to get through the treatments.

It still took every ounce of courage I had to show up for treatment at the appointed hour. On treatment days, the minute I opened my eyes I began to cry. There was no way out. It was another routine of "slam me to the mat and then try to help me back up again." I would pray for strength just before leaving the house. One day when I arrived for treatment I was told, "We're too busy to take you; come back later." I couldn't believe what I heard. I vowed they would never see me again. Does anyone but another cancer patient understand the trauma experienced by just submitting to treatment?

I went home and cut the grass to work off my frustration with the situation. A friend saw me in the yard and stopped in. She took me to the clinic later. Her care, my fierce determination, and my belief that the gain of chemo would be greater than the damage it caused, brought me back that day. Later, I understood there are different levels of need, and on that particular day at the clinic, there was a valid reason for telling me to come back later.

As I submitted to treatment, I prayed for a cure. If that wasn't possible, the next hope was for time, and if not a longer life, I hoped for quality time.

A caring doctor will always present information in a manner that is honest and supports the possibility of hope. One little bit of hope can turn people around. If a doctor does not offer hope, we need to find another doctor who will. Hope is an essential aspect of life and is crucial to life. We must never give up hope.

Cancer Truisms

1. You are not your disease.
2. Individuals are not statistics.
3. Doctors are mere mortals.
4. Diagnosis is an opinion, not a prediction.
5. Listen to your inner voice and go with it.
6. You determine how to respond to your disease.
7. Take charge of your illness. Participate.
8. Nothing is hopeless—never give up.
9. Nothing is forever—hang on for five minutes.
10. Believe treatment has great power.

*Show me your ways, Lord,
   teach me your path.*
                              —Psalm 25:4

~4~

Chemo—Strong Medicine

I have actually seen advances in treatment in the years between my two episodes of cancer. I learned that cancer is being detected earlier today because of new diagnostic techniques. Techniques for surgery and chemotherapy have improved dramatically. Diagnostic imaging provides clarity and detail that allows cancer specialists to make critical follow-up treatment decisions. As a result, mortality rates are falling for many common malignancies. The good news is that advances in cancer treatment are being made every day.

I can vouch for the fact, however, that conventional cancer therapy is toxic, painful, and dehumanizing. It is the use of strong medicines to destroy cancer cells. I learned that about a third of chemotherapy drugs are derivatives of natural sources, while others are created in the laboratory. Most of these agents are cellular poisons that interfere with a cell's ability to divide and grow. Since cancer cells divide faster than normal cells, they have a faster metabolic rate, taking a larger share of what comes to them in the bloodstream. In theory, the abnormal cells suffer more than the normal cells when these drugs are administered.

Cancer is a disease of our age, not just one disease, but many. My research revealed it is a catch-all name for several hundred different diseases with one thing in common—uncontrolled cell growth. We used to think of cancer as something that just happened to a person, and sometimes I still think it is random. I also now understand cancer as a long process. It is not something that happens instantaneously. Although cancer occasionally runs in families, a predisposition is what's inherited. The most significant risk factor in cancer is aging. As our bodies age, we are more susceptible to malignancies.

Further, I learned from my research that in some cancers, the chemotherapy is curative, while in others it weakens the cancer and allows the immune system a chance to overcome it. Because immune cells are also rapidly dividing cells, they frequently suffer the negative effects of chemotherapy. Chemo lowers the resistance to disease because the white blood cells of the immune system are destroyed. There were many days when I could not leave the house during treatment because my white cell count was so low that I was at risk of contracting something as seemingly insignificant as a cold. With a compromised immune system, a cold could kill. I submitted to routine blood tests each week during treatment, and immediately following treatment I would endure painful shots designed to rebuild my immune system.

Information is crucial. I wanted to know about the purpose and side effects of any drug proposed for me. I also wanted to know if there were alternatives to each test or treatment. As patients, we have the right to know and to refuse. We also have the right to see our charts, as well as to read our medical records including lab reports and x-rays. Hospitals and doctors have traditionally withheld records from patients. In 1984 the American Medical Association advised physicians to make records available upon patient request. If you want to see your records, ask. I noticed that I was never left alone in an exam room with my chart.

I know the goal of chemotherapy is to alter the cancer cells without harming healthy cells.

Faith, Hope, and Cancer

When reading the descriptions and warnings, it is difficult to agree to treatment. It seems like a terrible bargain to make—accepting poisons in order to survive. I had to trust God and the medical personnel. I was very nervous about treatment. After much thought and prayer, it became a matter of what the drugs could do *for* me—not *to* me.

    The scariest thing for me initially was the cramped chemo room. There were four chairs and two tables. Two patients would share a small tray table where drug bags had been deposited for administration. These bags were not marked. It was bad enough just being there for treatment without the concern that I might be given someone else's drugs. I was very nervous about it and did speak up at a cancer support meeting. Following that meeting, the bags were marked with the name of the individual patient along with the type of drug. It was a great relief to me. I made a difference for cancer patients receiving services at that clinic. I knew I couldn't presume the worst and had to remain positive, but it was tough going.

    My daughter stayed with me for the first treatment in 1996. Almost immediately, canker sores developed in my mouth. They made eating almost impossible. One of my friends came to the rescue by showing up at my door with home-baked custard for me. What a treat that was, and it was just the beginning of many good things she and others delivered to me. Within months, I lost my sense of taste and smell. I have never fully regained those two senses.

My enlarged lymph nodes went down immediately with the first treatment, as the oncologist said they would. It was encouraging. However, the tumor did not shrink after the second treatment. I reported this to my oncologist. The combination of drugs that made up the protocol was changed. During this process I discovered I could not tolerate the drug prednisone. I proceeded to wean myself off of it and reported this to the oncology nurse. She angrily informed me, "You need to learn how to follow directions." My response was, "No, you need to learn to listen to your patients." She was the gatekeeper doing her job; meanwhile, I needed a straight-jacket to handle my response to that drug.

In 1996, following each chemo treatment, I was given a shot every day for seven days to rebuild my white cells. By 2002, there was a new drug for this purpose. One injection of the new drug was apparently as powerful as seven shots of the original drug. During the second bout of treatments immediately following chemo,

I received one shot of the new drug and was unable to leave my bedroom for days. I was so weak and had so much bone pain I had to crawl to the bathroom as I could barely walk. I dubbed that drug "New Blasta," as it went off like a bomb in my body within an hour. In addition, another ugly side effect I experienced was colored lights shooting from the corners of my eyes, making it impossible to focus, let alone read, or do anything else for that matter. It was frightening. I refused that drug in remaining treatments. To this day, I occasionally experience the colored lights.

Once a port was installed in my chest in 2002, it too became a stressor to me. Every week it was used to draw blood samples. I was ever aware of its presence in my chest. I was told I could do any physical thing I wanted, so I never let it stop me from working in my yard. However, every little twinge in my chest would set off alarms in my mind. I was apprehensive about it, and that added to my stress level. Actually, just driving to the clinic I would experience anxiety. Following blood tests, I couldn't get out of there fast enough. It was hard to rest properly at night. I prayed often. I longed for my freedom.

When I finished chemo treatments in 2003, I was offered a new drug which would be administered twice a year as a preventative measure. Medical science is heavily involved in this antibody approach to treatment. My research indicated it was costly, but that was just one factor in the equation. I asked if there was another patient receiving this treatment who would be willing to talk with me about it. My name was provided to another patient who called me and we spoke in depth. This patient was in a different place in life than I was—much younger and praying for a bright future, including a family. While the treatment was described as brutal, she was willing to take it on. She helped me make my decision. It was one of the hardest decisions of my life. After much prayer, I rejected this treatment. It is in God's hands now.

    To make it through this period of my life, I would often look ahead to something happy to do the next day, something simple like browsing in a book store, working in my flowers, or walking my dog on the beach. All were great escapes. It was very difficult to go on with the endless treatment routines. I actually bribed myself just to continue the treatments. My idea was to buy myself a gift prior to each treatment, thereby ensuring that I would earn that reward by showing up for treatment. Sometimes the reward was simple and sometimes extravagant. Since I already had the gift—the first one was a lovely framed print—I felt obligated to appear at the clinic at the appointed hour. That idea worked for me. Shortly before the final treatment, I paid $37 for a fabulous bottle of hand lotion and never blinked an eye. Small comforts help ease large sorrows. I told myself, "You are one brave individual! Reward yourself! Take a bow!"

My brother and sister-in-law gave me the biggest reward of my life when I learned I was in remission. It was a seven-day Hawaiian cruise that docked at four different islands. It was a special celebration of life. The climate, the lush beauty of the islands, the scenery, fresh produce, particularly the fruits, all combined to make it a dream trip. It was certainly the most generous and most unexpected gift I have ever received. It was a brief glimpse of paradise. Everyone should have a caring brother like I do.

~II~

We Can Cope

Surely God is my salvation;
I will trust and not be afraid.
—Isaiah 12:2

~5~

Fight for Life

If you are a new cancer patient I can relate to how frightened you may be feeling. I know the heavy heart and the brain that can't be turned off. You probably never expected this to happen to you because we tend to think it only happens to others. You likely have a million questions one minute and are speechless the next. You may feel as if you have just been run over by a train. You may be wondering if there is any hope for recovery, or if you have a future. You are probably asking some of the same questions I did, "How much time do I have?" That's the question for months. I felt like I was on very shaky ground and was certain of nothing. Are you thinking you will never smile, laugh, or dream dreams one more time? Cancer can be overwhelming and seem too much to bear.

I ache for you and what you are experiencing. Take heart; you can get beyond this point. You can focus on hope and healing in the here and now.

Diagnosis is an opinion, not a prediction. What it will mean remains to be seen. We need to be careful how we think, because our lives are shaped by our thoughts. We need to cancel negative thoughts and try to think positively. For me it worked to narrow my focus and drop out of the world for a while. I had to find the courage to follow my heart and intuition. If you need time, take time. It's okay! One morning you may wake up recovered from cancer and see each new day as a miracle. You may learn that you can be well, even if not cured. Every day can be a victory, even if it's not an easy trip.

There is great reassurance in knowing others have survived cancer. When we are ill or facing adversity, we can begin the work of healing by following the path others have taken. My family history with cancer taught me a lot about surviving. My father was very calm, brave, and analytical when diagnosed. He even predicted how his death would affect his daughter and each of his sons. My mother, a very practical person, was also calm and brave when she learned of her illness. They were both excellent role models.

Fight for Life

They were strong people who fought for their lives to the end.

How do we prepare for the fight of our lives? The first step is to learn everything there is to know about the situation. This will empower us to change it. My bottom line was that no one knew what my future would be. However, I was more likely to have a future if I was prepared to fight for it. It is a profound theory. A strong positive attitude will create more miracles than the treatment itself.

I wanted to learn how other people coped with this disease, so I hung out at the library in 1996. I was looking for words of wisdom from anyone who had been there before me. Although I found many books on cancer, the library shelves held few personal accounts. I read Gilda Radner's story. Her courage and determination were admirable as she fought for, but eventually lost, her life. My stage IV diagnosis did not leave a lot of hope for me. I read the statistics and knew the survival rates. I asked myself, "Why can't I be in the percentage that survives?" I have no idea where that question came from, but it stuck with me. "Why can't I?"

The book of Job is about a man who looked tragedy in the face and said, "I'm going to live." It takes courage to choose this path. How I longed to shake myself free from the total concentration my disease-wracked body demanded. There was no way to do that. Ultimately, illness was always at the forefront of my mind and helped me fight. I too chose to live.

At one particularly low point in my treatment during the second bout with cancer, I recorded a scream in my journal. This was following a phone call regarding my white counts. I was packing away Christmas ornaments, and I had screamed out for no one to hear, "I want my life back!" I couldn't take it any more. The chemo had zapped every ounce of strength and courage from me. My white counts were so low they barely registered. The nurse who had called didn't want to give the numbers, saying instead, "They are low." I pressed for the numbers and received a sheepish, "They are very low," followed by, "They are very, very low." Finally, she gave me the numbers! There was nothing left to fight with. I was totally depleted.

There are no instant fixes to major medical problems or to tragedy in our lives. A patient's discussion of his or her condition with an oncologist will likely draw out few details. No one ever mentioned I might look like a prisoner of war shortly after my first treatment. I recall attending a management conference where I was approached by a co-worker from another area of the state. He asked, "Carol, what happened?" He said he didn't recognize me until he heard my voice. The story of cancer was told by my loss of hair, the look of devastation on my face, and the sadness reflected in my eyes. Even my body moved differently. My knees didn't want to work. My hands and feet were numb. Enter the fog. On two different occasions while driving my car close to home, I literally did not know where I was. Nothing was familiar. Panic washed over me. That situation called for instant prayer, "God, help me!" Regardless of how easy the oncologist might make it sound, treatment is no easy feat.

Serious illness involves tandem teamwork between the physician and the patient. Hopefully both tap into all their physical and spiritual resources to assist in the fight for life. Once I made the commitment to fight, I understood the most important resources were both spiritual and human. Sometimes it takes an illness or a tragedy in our lives to understand we are capable of resourcefulness and strength we never imagined we had.

In comparing my two journals from the first and second episode, I found I was even angrier in episode two. The first journal dealt with the physical aspects of the disease. It chronicled what was occurring within my body every single day as I continued working. The second journal was much more emotional and personal. It started with, "God be with me!" I was much less naïve and amazingly more candid the second time around. I unleashed raw emotions stemming from my great disappointment with the recurrence, which put me back to square one in all its horror. I felt as if I were letting so many people down. I couldn't imagine having to ask my friends and family to nurse me once again.

If you have cancer, don't be afraid to say so. Calling any disease by its name proves there is knowledge about it—something can be done about it. Initially, I could barely say the word out loud. But I soon realized that the more I said it, the easier it became for me. To some, cancer implies death. It is not a death sentence. While it is hard to believe at the time of diagnosis, it can become a life enhancer for some people. However, only in hindsight could that become clear. It's difficult, but we can try to see illness as an opportunity.

Yet, at the same time, I recognized the recurrence as a God moment and knew I was getting another chance. What lessons were just ahead? I prayed for the wisdom to understand what I was to learn. I told God I couldn't do this myself. I do believe we are called to live our lives the way we would if we knew with certainty that death was imminent. Everyone must work through individual feelings about death in his or her own good time. I urge you to never give up. Grab on with all that is within you. If, like me, you come out on the other end with remission, then rejoice! It's almost as good as a cure. We will benefit in two ways. It helps us take better care of our health and it allows us time to plan more realistically.

But those who hope in the Lord,
will renew their strength.
—Isaiah 40:31

~6~

No Passive Victims

Isn't it just common sense to be an activist patient? After all is said and done, no one cares more about the outcome of our treatment than we do. Knowledge and understanding is basic to empowerment. Being empowered permits us to participate in decisions and allows us some sense of control. A little assertiveness will go a long way. I decided if I was to beat this disease, I could not be a passive victim. I needed to be a part of my own treatment plan.

I refuse to submit to the role of victim or any role others determine to be my fate. I believe God alone gives life; God alone ends that life. Cancer is a problem to be corrected. Illness and injury are insulting and have the power to shatter self-image, but I am still the same, capable person. I do whatever it takes to keep going. I am prepared to state my needs and to ask questions. I expect to hear the information requested to make informed decisions. I intend to participate in my recovery. Life is not always easy. I learned to create strategies to deal with the turbulence of life.

My oncologist has a habit of making every procedure sound simple, fast and easy. No way! Please, just the facts will do. I have called him on this, and he good-naturedly jokes about it with me. I trust, respect, and like this man immensely. Further, one glance around his busy waiting room is enough to make me offer up a prayer of thanks for his expertise, thoroughness, and his gift of healing.

Any time I am scheduled for major lab tests, I inform the technician what type of needle to use. This isn't about power, but practicality. I also have a "three-stick tolerance." If a tech pokes me three times and still has not found a vein, I want another tech. I am assertive enough to inform them nicely of my three-stick rule. I fully appreciate and will never forget a man named Patrick who told me he would stick me once, and he would not hurt me in preparation for a PET scan. That is just what he did. It can be done.

Health care providers occasionally send questionnaires regarding customer service. I have always completed and returned them. I have noted customer service as an area where much improvement is needed. Medical people seem to forget that we are ultimately in charge of our health. We have the right to say "no" to anything. If we ask a question, we need an answer. Information should never be withheld from us.

I recall a confrontational scene with a nurse who refused to tell me why another blood test was necessary when seven tubes had been drawn the previous day. "You need it," was her repeated refrain. I have a great need to understand what is happening in my body. So, after five verses of this song, the conversation came to a screeching halt when I calmly used the F-word along with, "No more blood tests." Then, I got an explanation—and had the blood test. Why did such a simple thing have to reach such an extreme conclusion?

I am not recommending the use of that word despite how effective it was. I am still embarrassed about my crude language, and I did apologize to my oncologist. He was very generous and said he understood my frustration. The nurses joked with me about it for months. It became an inside joke and they were quick to inform me when checking in, "No blood tests today!" I include this story only to illustrate that literally anyone can be pushed over the edge when already in a precarious state of mind.

I advise you to know your hospital before you ever enter it. Granted, there are emergency situations where this would not be possible. Further, our choices are often limited to particular hospitals where particular physicians practice. Word-of-mouth and the personal experiences of friends and neighbors will provide fairly reliable information about the service one can expect to receive. It would be wise to check online at the hospital's Web site to gain information regarding practices and services offered. If hospital choices are available, consider visiting the actual sites to gain additional information. Another choice would be to request information from anyone working in the medical field. It is imperative that we arm ourselves with knowledge.

Upon entering a hospital for treatment, we are given consent forms to sign. It is wise to read the forms carefully and be aware of the risks. It is also important to ask questions if the forms are difficult to understand. All surgery is risky. Any invasive procedure can be complicated by one or more adverse outcomes. The goal is to get out of the hospital as quickly and as healthy as possible.

As patients we can fall victim to seemingly random risks. It happened to me. I was hospitalized for out-patient surgery to have a port installed in my chest for use during my second bout with cancer. I was informed immediately prior to surgery that there was a one percent chance that my lung could be punctured. It happened during the operation. An observant nurse alerted the surgeon that I was grimacing and should not be feeling pain. The collapsed lung was incredibly painful and was made even more so when a chest tube was inserted to drain fluids. I had a very bad night, and it would have been even worse without the help of close friends. Their support was a lifeline to me. One stayed overnight and was at my side the whole time.

That's when I realized how helpful it would be to have an advocate—someone to speak for us when we are hospitalized. We can ask a friend or family member to act on our behalf with doctors, nurses, or other staff. Following surgery, we are not alert to what is going on around us. An advocate can see that our needs are met and our questions answered. An advocate can keep a notebook of tests, procedures, results, and prescriptions. These records will come in handy later when attempting to make sense of the hospital bill. Having an advocate can help minimize potential problems.

I had no concept of the insurance wars I would encounter beginning in 1996. The insurance industry now requires claimants to work very hard to ensure payment. Each year, millions of workers in company-sponsored health plans face another cycle of higher premiums, co-payments and deductibles. The average patient knows very little about health. We are in the dark about the human body and why it gets sick. As a result of managed care, it seems to me that the average patient receives average care. When it comes to buying practically everything else in life, consumers have many options. That is not the case when it comes to health care.

To save time and frustration, it is always a good idea to review insurance coverage prior to treatment. It's important to determine if pre-approval is required by a particular plan. We can determine what procedures are covered and not covered, such as pre-existing conditions, elective surgery, or experimental procedures. Insurance is a business designed to generate profits. Health care is a huge profit-making machine.

It has been my experience that insurance companies frequently delay payments, claiming incorrect billing codes for a particular procedure. With services and procedures reduced to computer codes, one keystroke error by a data-entry clerk can turn a small charge into a huge fee. It's a good idea to maintain a journal or calendar noting services received. It takes a lot of energy to do this but it is worthwhile. A keystroke error in an account number can tie records up for months. How do they explain denying a service when they covered the same procedure months earlier? They don't!

Insurance forms are intricate; doctors and nurses are very busy. However, the patient's time is also valuable. It's best to review bills as soon as possible when they arrive and to keep all medical bills together. Sometimes consumers still find it virtually impossible to verify the accuracy of the charges. Even the most organized people can easily become frustrated. When calling my insurance company, much time was wasted while on hold. When I finally reached live people, they did not extend themselves in any way to help resolve my issues. I had to do the legwork myself. In some cases I felt like giving up and letting them off the hook. I also felt I was running in circles as I was told to call the health care provider, who in turn told me to call my insurance carrier. It seemed like a blame game designed to delay payment as long as possible. It happened many times, all when I was totally depleted from medical treatment. I had to hang in there and not give up.

The first denial of a claim is not the final answer. Persistence is key. I am very familiar with mystery bills listing charges from doctors I didn't even see. The biggest offenders in my experience were pathologists. Their offices were located in other cities or in neighboring states. They were unreachable and not concerned with my financial situation. Payment was their goal. They did not hesitate to forward my perceived bill to a collection agency with no warning to me. I did not owe them money and had to enlist the help of my employer's insurance specialist to get this issue resolved.

In 1997 my insurance carrier was changed, which is common practice with my former employer. Early in the coverage year I had a CT scan, which is costly. The new insurance carrier refused to pay for this test. The back-and-forth dragged on for months and then they demanded I drive to a city on the opposite side of the state for a hearing. I responded in writing, requesting a telephone hearing, which they finally agreed to. Six people plus corporate counsel were introduced to me over the phone. I had done my homework and was prepared to make a case because the CT scan was a service I was entitled to. As a result, the claim was covered.

My best advice is to work closely with the insurance staff in the medical building where services are provided. It's important to get to know them. They should be allies in this war, as the common goal is payment for services. The carrier's health care cost information is available on the Internet for quick review. In some cases it is most helpful to contact the human resource department maintained by employers to provide additional information regarding the coverage offered. This can be critical in resolving insurance issues. I would recommend contacting state insurance commissioners if something seems amiss.

For links to state insurance departments, go to www.naic.org and click on your state of residence, then click on "Consumer," and then click on "Fraud reporting" or "Filing a complaint." Insurance issues can be a continuing struggle and source of frustration.

*Come to me, all who are weary and burdened,
and I will give you rest.*
                              —Matthew 11:28

~7~

Does Anyone Care?

I needed to know that someone cared. To me, caring means being there. What prompted me to write this book was the death of my first great-grandchild in 2003. Sweet baby Alyssa appeared to be healthy when she was born, but only lived 16 hours. I watched my granddaughter and her husband deal with the trauma of her birth and death, and their overwhelming grief, while close friends and family remained remote and silent. Uncertain what to say, people often unintentionally offend or hurt loved ones. It is amazing to me how many people will say, months, even years later, they didn't know what to say, so they said nothing.

This is about connection to people in our lives, about friendship and caring, and so it is about love.

Our lives are made up of a variety of relationships, and all of them are based on communication. One little word can make a tremendous difference in someone's life. All interaction is dependent on our ability to speak with and understand each other. We communicate on many different levels at the same time. Only a small percentage is verbal; words have power, but actions speak louder than words. The larger percentage of communication is nonverbal. We need to use our ears, eyes, and even our hearts to fully understand one another. We need to listen with our ears, but understand with our hearts.

We also communicate through touch. Touch is very powerful. "Reach out and touch someone" is not just an advertising slogan. Touch is so meaningful to the patient. If a visitor asks me, "Can I hug you?" I will say yes, without hesitation, every time. During the course of my illness, people told me, "I feel so helpless; I can't think of anything to say or do." Their presence, phone calls, and e-mails were all encouraging and important to me. The words can be simple. A pure statement of their thoughts is always right.

I believe the most basic and powerful way to connect with another is to listen. I find there are very few good listeners in the world. Listening is a great gift. It implies mutual respect. Sometimes, as patients, we need to talk about what we are afraid of. We do not necessarily want answers to our problems. We simply need to release our thoughts. We need a sounding board. It's important that we are allowed to talk. A person who is listened to feels cared about. The only exception is the patient who is not ready to talk. That position must be honored.

Many people dealing with illness experience objective clarity about their lives. Their perspective on life has changed dramatically. As patients we may feel temporarily detached from life. Our lives have taken a sharp turn, have fallen apart abruptly. The unthinkable has happened. We still need to know if anyone is listening and if anyone cares. I vividly recall one of my co-workers coming to me immediately after a meeting at which I announced my retirement. She followed me out, and inquired, "It's bad, isn't it?" We hugged and both cried. Her empathetic and understanding gesture touched my heart.

Hopefully, there are stashes of love and understanding waiting to help us stand on our own two feet again. Good friends sustain one another. They show up when it matters most—and even when it doesn't. I appreciate my friends and am grateful they are in my life. Among my closest friends are my oldest ones, but I would never discount my connection to new friends.

Faith, Hope, and Cancer

In 1996 I had a long conversation with an old friend, who was a cancer survivor, about my upcoming final chemo treatment. I expressed doubts about my body's ability to tolerate another treatment. My total health had been in a downward spiral as treatment went on. My friend instantly announced she would be taking me for treatment. She made sure I saw it through to the end. It was a three-hour drive for her each way. She did it for me because she cared.

It is only with the heart that we can see clearly. We need to get out of our heads and into our hearts. When we speak from the heart, our words can touch the heart of the receiver. The words can be simple. A pure statement of what we are feeling is always right. The most important thing we ever give others is our attention—especially when given from the heart. It's all about sensitivity to others. Caring is even more important than the spoken message. Just being there is enough. It costs nothing to give someone hope. It's free!

Friends are crucial to our well-being. I believe no one is in our lives by accident. The support of friends has been linked to a hardier immune system, fewer illnesses, and improved odds of surviving illness. A friend is often the only person to give us the reality check we need. There is enormous power in the simplest of human relationships. In order to be as healthy as we can be, we need social interaction. As patients, we also need encouragement to get beyond illness.

Good people skills are important. Jesus gave us the golden rule, "Do unto others as you would have them do unto you." If we put ourselves in someone else's shoes, we will automatically show more consideration, patience, and kindness. We also learn truths about ourselves in the process. The patient does not need sympathy, nor does the patient want pity; the patient does need empathy, help, and support. Empathy meets two fundamental needs: the need to be understood, and the need to have feelings validated. An empathetic attitude greatly enhances our ability to get along with people. As a bonus, when focusing on the other person, we forget about ourselves.

We are all part of each other's reality. We are all connected to one another. We need to be aware of our influence on others or how our attitudes could potentially affect them. The power of the experts, particularly the doctors, is tremendous. The way in which an expert sees us may easily become the way in which we see ourselves. If the patient is seen as a hopeless case, that same attitude can quickly be transferred, thereby causing the patient to lose faith in the recovery process. We need to ask the experts for the truth, but always look for the positives.

We can so easily hurt others. There were several scenarios I found disturbing after the word was out about my illness. Some co-workers seemed to be uncomfortable around me. I felt invisible at times or perhaps contagious. Maybe they thought I had lost my mind, or just my hearing. More than once people started speaking very deliberately and loudly to me, as if I were deaf.

As a cancer patient, I craved normalcy and the same ordinary things I had experienced prior to my diagnosis. I did not want to be isolated. It takes incredible courage to live through a serious illness. I found I could do it, but only with a lot of help. I wanted to go on living with a sense of purpose. I needed encouragement. For the most part, I realized I was right where I was supposed to be, even though I didn't understand God's plan for me. I needed to remain grounded in the real world while undergoing treatments. My attitude was helped immensely by prayers, good wishes, and a goal of returning to normal routines and activities. As a patient, what did I hold on to? I know God was holding on to me, and that is all I needed to know to find peace of mind.

Friends are free to come and go. Not all friendships last forever. I had friends drop out of my life upon learning of my cancer. It hurt. Illness may end marginal friendships. Occasionally people will disappear when most needed. It is hard to forget rejection, but we need to let it go. We have more important issues to deal with. I found great comfort in the family and friends who stepped forward when there was nothing left to be said. People cannot fully understand what the patient has endured unless they have been there themselves. But their presence says it all. It says they care!

All caregivers can do is try to understand the fears and insecurities common to people facing serious illness. As a cancer patient I found many kinds of support meant a great deal to me. I know life is full of chores and obligations. It is not always easy to take time from busy schedules to meet the needs of others. To hold someone's hand, hug someone, or just pat someone on the shoulder is a blessing. It is offering God's healing touch. What a powerful thought!

As friends or caregivers, if you are unable to visit the patient and choose to write instead, it's best to do so as soon as possible. Putting if off makes it more difficult. Get well cards and letters are always special. A sincere sentence speaks loudly. It helps to say what you feel—if you're upset, you can say so. If you don't know what to say, you can say that. Telephone and e-mails are a quick, easy way to show support, care, and concern. It's important because patients might feel as if they have been abandoned or written off. They might find themselves excluded from social activities and things they care about. If people you are close to become ill, you must not desert them.

How Can You Help?

1. Be available.
2. Don't treat me any differently.
3. Let me talk.
4. Give the gift of friendship.
5. Offer encouragement.
6. Stay in touch.
7. Be authentic. Be yourself.
8. Pray for me. It will help both of us.
9. Don't abandon me.
10. Offer hugs and companionship.

When visiting, it's best to follow the lead of the patient, but show interest. As a patient, I didn't want to be flattered or told how wonderful I looked. I already knew how I looked, and it was anything but good. If anyone asked how I was, and I responded with the automatic "Fine," I wanted them to accept that answer. Often I was pressed for details with a quizzical "Really?" Stop already with the questions! I was doing the best I could at the time. I always needed to process information about my condition before discussing it with others.

When the patient knows that someone is interested, conversation will develop naturally. It's okay to begin with simple comments such as, "I'm sorry to hear that you are ill," and wait for a response. How tough is that? There is no one right thing to say. Each conversation is unique. If we speak of good times from the past, it shows caring about the friendship. We can trust in the relationship to see us both through the hard times. We can start talking with each other. We can laugh together or just share.

When visiting, it is more than acceptable to cry. There is great strength and courage in tears. Shedding tears in the presence of a loved one shows trust. We don't cry tears for them, but rather with them. Tears are a gift of grace. Holding back tears takes a great deal of energy. That energy could be better used just talking with each other. It's sometimes good to bring a book and read to the patient, if that would be enjoyable. A chapter or two is enough. We can let the patient know that we are available for phone calls. There are many different ways for us to help out. If we say, "Call me if you need anything," chances are good that call would never be made. Better questions to ask are: "What do you need?" or "What can I do?"

A great pick-me-up to anyone's spirit is to receive flowers or encouraging messages. A single rose is a perfect gift. We can also help by cooking dinner, providing comfort food, cleaning the house, babysitting or picking kids up after school, running errands, or grocery shopping. We can try to anticipate the needs of the patient. The list is endless. These thoughtful gestures will be appreciated and long remembered.

When visiting patients in the hospital, we need to remember they are there because they are ill and require special care. Visiting should be postponed when patients are napping. Their quiet time should be respected. A note left behind will let them know they had a visitor.

Know Before You Go

1. If sick, stay home. Patients have impaired immune systems.
2. Wash your hands before visiting.
3. Stay off of the bed.
4. Don't bring your small children along.
5. Do not smoke before your visit, as the odor lingers on clothing.
6. Limit the length of your visit. Be aware of the patient's condition.
7. If the patient already has visitors, it's not a good time to visit.
8. Do not waken a patient just for a visit.
9. Don't ask to use the patient's bathroom.
10. Ask if there is anything you can do for the patient right now.

What Not to Say to the Patient

1. "I know exactly how you feel." (No, you don't have a clue.)
2. "God never gives you more than you can handle." (That's arguable.)
3. "Think on the bright side—you don't have to go to work." (Most people would prefer working to being ill.)
4. "You'll be on your feet in no time." (I'm not sure about that.)
5. "You are a very strong person!" (I never felt so vulnerable.)
6. Do not tell horror stories of other patients. (I have no need to know.)
7. Many people are sensitive to what they perceive as pity.
8. Avoid any attempts at nervous jokes. They are seldom funny and indicate you care more about your comfort than the patient's.
9. Don't criticize the patient's doctor, the hospital, or the staff.
10. Refrain from offering advice. (You have no medical expertise.)

Rejoice with those who rejoice;
mourn with those who mourn.
Live in harmony with one another.
—Romans 12:15–16

~8~

Prayer and People

Many people have asked me, "What do you know about getting well?" My simple answer is prayer and people, or people praying for me. It's about a strong support system. It's about the people in that system and their willingness to go the distance with me. Healing is not magic and it is more than using the right formula. With help from many people, I made an active decision to fight for my life and to never give up hope.

Healing takes on many forms, and all individuals heal in their own unique ways. Of course there are many contributing factors to remission, but I feel that the single most important one is people praying. Prayer was the key to my remission in both the first and second bouts. Although I live in the upper Midwest, I was told prayer chains on both the east and west coasts prayed for me. I loved that encouragement. My name was also submitted several times to the Mormon Tabernacle for prayer. The mail brought me countless messages of hope from across the country. I know the prayers were offered every day. My strongest weapon was prayer.

My parish prayed for me. My minister was just one of the spiritual resources available to me. Others included the parish nurse, a wonderful friend who also assigned a trained Stephen Ministry volunteer to meet with me each week. This special person was a great help and comfort to me. We were in similar occupations, and connected immediately. The purpose of the Stephen Ministry program is not to solve problems, but to provide a listener as issues of vital importance are discussed confidentially. It is an extension of the church's caring ministry to its members. I truly believe when there is a need the Lord will provide. How very fortunate I was to work with someone who allowed me to express myself at a time when I needed to talk.

I initiated a monthly meeting with a licensed clinical psychologist. This person had spent years counseling cancer patients. She was very bright and very caring. I met with her during my treatment for both the first and second bouts with cancer. I cannot thank her enough for her caretaking and words of wisdom. This very qualified individual gave tremendous help by allowing me to clarify my thoughts and encouraging me to make my own decisions. Early in my treatment series in 1996, I met with her at 7 a.m. prior to a chemo treatment scheduled later that day. I told her I would be a no-show. I simply could not tolerate the drug prednisone, which was part of my protocol. When taking it I felt totally out of control. I described my extreme reaction to that drug and how I had weaned myself off of it. I refused to ever take it again.

Once she heard my predicament she reached for the telephone and dialed the clinic, getting an instant response. I can still hear her, "This is Dr. J, and I need to talk to Dr. Ed." What an impressive little dynamo! She then handed me the phone to explain to my oncologist what I had just told her. He listened carefully, and then assured me he would use another drug. He gently told me I must not delay my treatment. That problem was solved, thanks to her intervention.

How did I get well? My faith in God and my understanding that, in the best of times and the worst of times, it is people who sustain us and see us through whatever life is serving up. I credit my immediate family, my friends, and my neighbors for the very strong support system they were for me. They were continually looking out for and checking in on me.

I also credit excellent medical care and am very grateful for all the dedicated medical professionals working with me. I admit it took a while for us to understand each other, but at some point the nurses realized that I did not ask frivolous questions. It became easier to get answers. I have great respect for the doctors and nurses who work with cancer patients. They are special people, and it must be incredibly difficult work.

The role of prayer and medicine has been questioned and debated forever. Faith and medicine have been combined since the beginning of time. A *USA Weekend* poll revealed more than 75 percent of adults believe spirituality and prayer can help them recover from illness or injury. The evidence that prayer helps healing is not only anecdotal but can be measured scientifically. Medical journals are full of studies proving the power of prayer. I can attest to receiving help every time I ask for it.

My Resources for Getting Well

1. Prayer
2. Support of family and friends
3. Parish staff support
4. A trusted oncologist
5. Counselors and support groups
6. Chemotherapy
7. Alternative methods
8. Research and reading independently
9. Participation in my own care
10. Faith, hope, and love

~III~

I Will Survive

*Trust in the Lord with all your heart,
And lean not on your own understanding.*
—Proverbs 3:5

~9~

Build on Success

There is a lot to be said for previous successes. Positive experiences from our past build confidence at any time, but especially when we are ill. Thinking about the winning events in life can help. For me, the thought of *I beat polio; I can beat cancer*, was like a drumbeat. It replayed in my head throughout my cancer episodes. I didn't totally beat polio, but have led a fairly normal life with few restrictions on my physical abilities.

I contracted polio in 1940. I have thought about its impact on my life, and it was a defining event. I was very fortunate to thrive following it. I have constant reminders that my life is not as easy as that of others. However, the polio experience reinforced my ability to make the physical and emotional changes necessary for survival.

The challenges polio posed were important lessons. First, I learned about the reality of life. I also learned about discipline, which was encompassed in a strict exercise regimen, I followed for years. As a result, I understood I could rise to the occasion and fight the monsters of life. I knew from the day cancer was diagnosed I wasn't going down quietly. I would fight with everything I had.

Further, I recognize I did not survive polio alone. Many others believed in me, starting with my parents and extended family. They were strong people who had high expectations of me. The belief, love, and encouragement my family instilled in me gave me a positive attitude that can't be shaken to this day. I learned to succeed in whatever I was doing, but only with the support and help of others. I did not do it by myself. My early religious training taught me to count my blessings.

Thankfully, the polio epidemics are a nightmare from the past. More than two million now-middle-aged polio survivors were left with psychological scars from that experience. I was two years old when diagnosed with polio. My parents took me to a hospital many miles away for treatment. I have no distinct memories of that serious illness, but have heard favorite family stories about events that occurred during that period. An uncle loved to tell of his visit with me. Living in the community where the hospital was located, he purchased a doll. I was in isolation but he was allowed to observe as the nurse presented the doll to me. I immediately flung it out of the crib, screaming, "I want my mama!" At age two (the terrible twos) I innately knew what I needed—and it wasn't a doll.

I was required to exercise rigorously from age two until my teen years. I was followed routinely by doctors, tested and measured while my progress was charted over the years. I was never treated differently by my family, although many who suffered from this disease were ostracized and verbally abused. Some who contracted polio were even blamed for their disease because of a lack of information and education about it.

I do recall my father insisting that I take my meds—I still have trouble swallowing pills—and that I walk with a book on my head every day for twenty minutes to improve my posture. Every new pair of shoes went to the shoemaker to add a lift before I ever wore them—brown Oxfords I absolutely hated.

As I grew up, I discovered I could compete with my three brothers in sports. I could run just as fast and jump just as high as they could. My middle brother and I shared roller skates. We are still very close to this day.

Sports were a great distraction, and the spirit of competition was keen. At a recent family reunion I was remembered by second cousins as, "the little blonde girl who had polio."

There is a twist to this story. The polio virus did damage to my body many years ago while setting the stage for new symptoms that could trigger post-polio syndrome. Following the development of polio vaccines, polio was thought to be eradicated and stabilized. It was believed that once polio survivors recovered muscle strength, their physical abilities would remain for the rest of their lives. For unknown reasons, some people who survived polio decades ago entered a late phase of accelerated weakness and muscle shrinkage. Scientists do not know why. It is a frightening phenomenon. Although muscular weakness is common to all of us as we age, such weakness would be more pronounced in those who, like me, experienced the permanent weakness of polio.

Through the years, polio survivors developed new symptoms, which included muscle and joint pain, sleep disorders, heightened sensitivity to anesthesia and cold, along with difficulty in breathing and swallowing. I recognized my sensitivity to cold and anesthesia a long time ago.

First seek the counsel of the Lord.
—1 Kings 22:5

~10~

Ask the Experts

Feeling helpless is the worst thing for one's immune system. We are at the mercy of our bodies, but to whatever degree we can, we still direct them. I was willing to do almost anything to be healed. So I took my medications and my vitamins, slept when I could, and showed up for my treatments—no easy feat. I read constantly, searching for answers and personal accounts. The book, *Peace, Love and Healing,* by Bernie Siegel asks the question, "What are the benefits of having this disease?" I remember first reading it, and having a strong desire to throw the book into the fireplace. Was he crazy? I had trouble connecting the dots on this one, but months later when I did, I started reading everything he had written.

Bernie Siegel identified what he came to know as "exceptional patients" who refused to be victims, did not take anything for granted, armed themselves with information, and made their own decisions about treatment. These patients would fight if they had to, and had every intention of participating in their care. Their heads were held high. These people knew what they wanted and were prepared to ask for it.

I am in awe of this medical man who shaves his head to better relate to patients losing their hair during treatment. Another book titled *How to Live Between Office Visits* answered a question Dr. Siegel received many times over by simply stating, "You live your life one day at a time." Other books by Dr. Siegel are *Prescriptions for Living*, and *Love, Medicine and Miracles*.

Another writer who influenced my thinking was Dr. Andrew Weil with his understanding of ancient mind-body medicine. He has written many books. My favorites are *Spontaneous Healing, Eight Weeks to Optimum Health,* and *Eating Well for Optimum Health.* Dr. Weil advises cancer survivors to start with a plan for improving health and reducing future cancer risk. He devotes an entire chapter to that topic in the *Eating Well* book. As we increase our knowledge of diet, supplements, exercise, and mind-body connections, we almost certainly will decide to change some aspects of our lives.

Ask the Experts

In 1996 I had heard of a book called *A Cancer Battle Plan*. This book became a second Bible to me. There was so much good information in it. The author and her husband, Anne and David Frahm, present six strategies for beating cancer. The first strategy was to know your enemy; second was to cut off enemy supply lines; third was to rebuild your natural defense system; fourth was to bring in reinforcements; fifth was to maintain morale; and the sixth was to carefully select your professional help. This book offers a comprehensive nutritional program for all people. I frequently refer to this book when people ask me questions. It is one of the most-used books in my collection.

In 2002, *The Purpose-Driven Life* by Rick Warren was published and quickly became a bestseller. This book has answered so many of my questions and redirected my thinking about heaven as my eternal home. It clarified my belief that God knows what is best for my life; that life on earth is a trust, a temporary assignment, a classroom. This life is preparation for the next. It taught me that my life was never about me. I followed the author's advice to read one chapter a day for forty days to discover God's purpose for my life. I believe everyone can benefit from the timeless message of the word of God contained in this book. After several years I can still open it to any page and learn something more about myself and my mission. It is a quick and inspiring read.

In 2003 I discovered a book titled *Fighting Cancer From Within* by Martin L. Rossman. This is an excellent book on using the power of your mind for healing. He has also written a book on guided imagery for healing. I had practiced this technique in 1996 and believed it had great power. I was aware my tumor was shrinking following the very first chemo treatment. My questions, "Is it shrinking? Is it shrinking?" were nonstop as treatment progressed. It was very encouraging to me. I highly recommend this book for anyone diagnosed with cancer. It is not a book that needs to be read cover to cover, but is best used as a reference guide.

With the recurrence of cancer in 2002, I found Dr. Susan Lark, who is one of the foremost authorities in the fields of clinical nutrition and preventative medicine. She has written eleven books on women's health and healing. Lark writes a monthly newsletter to which I subscribe. Her special reports are loaded with essential information. Long, healthy lives are her goal. She addresses issues and provides complete explanations of chosen topics. One of particular interest to me was the acid/alkaline balance in the body. It is an important physiological function and yet rarely discussed. My interest was sparked as I was taking an "alkaline agent" prescription drug each day.

I believe in life-long learning, and I couldn't survive without the world of books, periodicals, and other educational sources. The library offers information on any subject, as well as entertainment and pure pleasure. I do not travel far in a car without popping in a book on tape and being entertained for hours. For me, there is no better therapy than getting lost in a book. Additionally, personal computers are available at the library, so anyone can access the Internet for research.

We can educate ourselves and take charge of our own healing. We have a choice, and the ability to analyze and access information that may improve our health. Knowledge is power. Technology allows instant access to information about illness. Many clinics or hospitals offer a patient library, which is a good place to start.

There are many reliable resources on the World Wide Web as well. The most useful Internet sites I found include:

- National Library of Medicine, which is found at www.nlm.nih.gov.

- International Cancer Information Center, found at www.cancer.gov/oma/hnc1b2.htm.

- National Cancer Institute at www.cancer.gov.

Good resources can also be found at www.WebMD.com and www.Medlineplus.gov.

Government health sites, such as the National Cancer Institute, as well as home pages for medical schools and associations, are loaded with useful information. Help is also available from the National Cancer Institute Cancer Information Service at (800) 422-6237.

NOTES

A merry heart does good like medicine.
—Proverbs 17:22

~11~

Options in Therapy

Cancer needs to be addressed at all levels: physical, mental, and spiritual. There are choices beyond traditional treatments. We need to explore all health options. Many of those options take advantage of natural healing mechanisms. We can think in terms of our potential for good health as being greater when we use more than a single approach. What do our bodies really need? They need proper rest, fresh air, exercise, good food, love, respect, and affection. If we are willing to meet those needs, we must also recognize that we live in a sea of carcinogens and have to protect ourselves. Chemotherapy and radiation are damaging to the immune system.

I do not like to take drugs. During treatment I refused many drugs that were offered to me in addition to chemotherapy. I have always been interested in natural products and remedies. My co-workers recommended a local naturopathic doctor who was building a very good reputation as a healer. What I like about naturopathy is the belief that the body has considerable power to heal itself. Naturopathic physicians are primarily teachers, educating and empowering patients to assume more personal responsibility for their health. For eight years I have worked together with a naturopathic doctor on a health-promoting program, and his willingness to answer all my questions was appreciated.

I recall the first step in this program was to detoxify my liver following chemotherapy treatments, both the first and second bouts. Chemo has a toxic effect on the body, especially the liver. I also learned about cleansing the colon twice a year, water purification, drinking green tea, and the vitamins and minerals I needed to pump up my immune system.

Complementary, alternative, integrative, New-Age medicine, holistic medicine, or even nontraditional medicine all encompass a trend away from drugs and surgery. The idea that outlook and mood are related to health is a central principle of alternative methods. A positive outlook in the face of serious illness is, in many cases, at least as important to health and resiliency as traditional medical treatment. There are many different therapies, so how do we know which ones might be right for us?

A complementary therapy refers to supportive methods that are used in addition to conventional medicine. Some therapies have been shown to help relieve symptoms and improve quality of life by lessening side effects of conventional treatments. These therapies may provide psychological and physical benefits to the patient. Good examples of this include acupuncture and massage.

Many methods can be safely used along with conventional treatment to help relieve symptoms or side effects, to ease pain, minimize stress, and to help us enjoy life more. Rule number one: investigate before buying or trying. The best approach is to look carefully at all the choices. It is important to check with a physician before trying a dietary supplement or a self-prescribed remedy rather than, or in addition to, prescription drugs.

Here is a list and brief description of options I read about and tried:

Affirmations
We can help heal our attitudes with affirmations. I listened to a Bernie Siegel affirmation audio tape while commuting to and from work. It was from his *Prescriptions for Living* series. Bernie presents affirmations by reading a statement, and the listener repeats it. The affirmations are stated as facts; you allow them into your mind and they become real. It goes like this: "You feel good about yourself." Response: "I feel good about..." "You let go of your negative thoughts." "I let go of my..." It is positive reinforcement about your health. Another idea is to write down a favorite affirmation and tape it onto a mirror and read it out loud every day. A positive attitude will develop as the message becomes part of who you are.

Counselor or support group
We are all wounded in life in some way. Most counseling clients just need a little help over the rough spots. Support groups bring people with similar issues together. They learn they are not alone and that others struggle with the same things. Many psychologists believe group therapy is extremely important in the patient's recovery.

People form support groups to share their pain and move forward. Participants can be more objective because they are strangers to each other. If we are upset about our situation, we need to get those emotions out. We need to open up, whether it is talking with friends about how we feel or writing each day in a journal. We will be happier and healthier if we do not hide our wounds.

When we join a group, we can help others and ourselves survive by sharing our stories. Various studies show patients who attended support group sessions survived longer than those not in a group. Support groups are commonly led by medical personnel. I joined a group and found it helpful for sharing my concerns.

Deep breathing

Breathing constitutes life. How we breathe reflects our health and how we feel about ourselves. Life-giving oxygen cleanses the bloodstream and energizes the whole body. Deep breathing ensures a good flow of oxygen into the lungs. Many people develop poor or incorrect breathing habits throughout their lives. To improve our breathing, we must first become aware of it. It is the key to calming mind and body. Our breathing becomes shallow and rapid when we are anxious, but slow and deep when we are at ease.

Breathing is an automatic, involuntary action, but it can be consciously controlled. In times of acute stress, taking a minute to slow down and control our breathing will calm us down instantly. Deeper breathing and a slower pulse are recognized signs of good health—the deeper the breath, the more body tissues can be oxygenated and the stronger the heart becomes. For more information see Dr. Andrew Weil's book, *Breathing*. To summarize the benefits: increased energy levels make exercise more efficient, muscle control is enhanced, valuable nutrients are distributed to vital tissues in the body, providing clearer thinking.

Exercise

We have the power to improve how we feel. Regular exercise frees the mind and body; it can improve mood, increase self-esteem, reduce anxiety, promote sleep, lower high blood pressure, and help weight loss. It doesn't have to involve a lot of time, joining a gym, or spending lots of money to become fit. As little as twenty minutes a day of walking can make a big difference in fitness levels. As a bonus, exercise dramatically reduces stress. In the long term, we can expect stronger bones and better balance, stronger hearts and bodies. We can find an activity that suits us. We need to know our limitations and not push our bodies too hard.

We can choose forms of exercise that easily fit into our lifestyle. In my case, I credit my golden retriever, Katy, with keeping me active because she kept me walking during my chemotherapy treatments. The cumulative side effects of chemo left my hands and feet numb, my joints painful and stiff, but Katy needed a walk every day, and that is what we did. The great thing about dogs is their acceptance of us without reservation. They are so attuned to our needs. If we need exercise, they get us moving. If we are sick, they sit quietly beside us, providing healing energy. They give unconditional love so freely. What a joy animals bring to our lives!

Laughter

We need to remember to laugh! It is good for the body, mind and soul. Norman Cousin's book, *Anatomy of an Illness,* tells how he recovered from a rare arthritic condition by laughing. He discovered a dose of belly laughs gave him two hours of pain relief. He called it internal jogging. Subsequent research shows there are many benefits to laughter. It can relax the whole body and it burns many more calories than one would in a resting state. There is also medical evidence that laughter produces more T-cells, an important part of the body's immune system. It may even stimulate the brain to produce endorphins which are the body's natural painkillers. Humor can lessen anxiety, lift depression, and raise tolerance for pain. The physiological effects on the body stimulate both the circulatory and the immune systems.

My co-workers were an important factor in my recovery. Staff kept me laughing by constantly pulling pranks and jokes on me. Turning my clock back an hour was one of their favorites. Notes or cartoons were always waiting for me. After I lost my hair, many of the conversations in my office began with "Now, don't flip your wig over this, but..." These situations helped me maintain normalcy. I could never repay the kindness shown me. So many people in so many ways helped me through the cancer experience.

We can find movies, audio and video tapes, and books to make us laugh. The Woody Allen quotes I had posted in my office kept me smiling each time I read them. My favorite is, "Ninety percent of success is just showing up." Another, "Life is filled with miserableness, unhappiness, loneliness and suffering—and it's over much too quickly." Laughter is the easiest therapy you will ever find.

Meditation

Meditation can bring relief by creating a feeling of peace and serenity. It can silence inner chatter and help you recognize and stop negative thoughts. It begins with relaxation and is a method of controlling the mind. Many people who practice meditation have improved their physical and mental well-being. Meditation can be for everyone, whatever their lifestyle. However, it was difficult for me because my mind tended to wander; over and over again it had to be brought back to the point of focus. It takes practice and may seem difficult at first. What helped me get started was doing it on a regular basis for just a few minutes at a time.

The most helpful thing is to find a quiet spot for relaxation. If we keep a place just for meditation, our brains will associate it with peaceful feelings, which puts us in the right state of mind to meditate. Meditation can help us think more clearly and improve our energy levels. It can also improve physical health because the mind has power to bring about change in the body.

Music therapy

Music therapy promotes healing by inspiring or relaxing its listeners. Research confirms that music bypasses the conscious mind. It goes directly to the part of the brain that controls emotions and vital pulses. Music can elevate moods, thus restoring hope and lifting spirits.

Music is a daily part of my life and I believe it contributed to my healing. Music therapy has been used in combination with medicine for hundreds of years. I have an eclectic taste in music and a large compact disc collection. I added to it when I was ill. I also tune into National Public Radio every morning for classical music, as I am hooked on it.

A formalized approach to music therapy first began in World War II when veterans' hospitals used music to treat soldiers suffering from shell shock. Scientific studies have shown the positive value of music therapy. A number of clinical trials have shown the benefit of music for relieving acute pain, including pain from cancer. Other trials revealed a reduction in heart rate, blood pressure, breathing rate, insomnia, depression, and anxiety with music therapy. No one knows exactly how music benefits the body, but it does distract the mind from focusing on pain, allowing people to forget their problems for a while.

Nutrition

When being treated for cancer, proper nourishment helps us feel better and is essential to our recovery. It helps the body fight disease by increasing chances of a favorable response to therapy. Good eating habits also make us less susceptible to infections that could weaken us. We need to do our homework to get the most from our diets. Powerhouse fruits and vegetables are packed with the most nutrients and antioxidants. These foods are easy to spot in the grocery store produce departments because of their intense colors. We need to eat our spinach.

Understanding basic nutrition can help speed our recovery. Optimum nutrition means eating the right food at the right time. Breakfast starts the metabolism, and the biggest meal of the day should be around noon, when the metabolism is most effective. It is best not to eat after eight o'clock at night.

Sleep

Sleep is a distinct state of mind and body. It is essential to our overall well-being. The body is at rest, the metabolism is lowered, and the mind is unconscious to the outside world. Sleep allows the body to repair and rejuvenate itself. A good night's sleep is like medicine. A deep rest allows the body to recover from fatigue and stress. It activates our own self-repair and balancing mechanisms.

Every time I had chemo I would come home and nap for an hour or two. Sleep was total oblivion, which was good for me, and it allowed me to escape temporarily. How much sleep an individual needs varies from one person to the next. A regular sleep routine is helpful, as is getting exercise during the day, and avoiding caffeine or alcohol three hours before bedtime.

Dreaming helps by sweeping stress and tension from the nervous system. We can function at our peak after a good night's sleep. It is important that we learn what helps us get the deepest and most refreshing rest possible. Sleep medications should be a last resort and used temporarily only when other strategies as mentioned above aren't working.

To learn more about how to maximize a night's sleep, go to www.sleepfoundation.org.

Visualization

A technique known as visual imagery fascinated me when I first read the book, *Getting Well Again,* by O. Carl Simonton. I decided immediately to try it. I had seen my tumor during the guided ultrasound biopsy. It was surrounded by colored flashing lights. The visualization process involves focusing on a specific image twice a day while imagining achieving a chosen goal. In my mind, I saw the elimination of my tumor as my T-cells did their job of shrinking it. The colored flashing lights dancing on the ultrasound screen represented the T-cells. My plan was to "turn out the lights." Not only did I practice the visualization, but I talked to my tumor as well. I told it, "Your lights are going out. I am shutting you down and I intend to win this battle."

Through visualization we can direct our healing to any area that requires care. By focusing on one area with the intention of bringing healing energy to it, we can potentially "think" away cancer or any other medical problem. Creative visualization calls on our inner healer.

Water

Water is one of our most critical nutrients. I drink plenty of water during the day. It is vital for good health and boosts the energy level. Each day, our bodies require an intake of over two quarts of water to function optimally. About one quart is provided in the foods we eat. This means we need to drink an additional quart of liquids a day to maintain good water balance. We don't ever want to allow ourselves to become dehydrated or we may suffer from a variety of symptoms including nausea, headache, and exhaustion. Not drinking enough liquids puts stress on the body.

An adequate intake of water will leave us feeling refreshed and more energetic. It also helps protect the kidneys and flushes toxins and other waste products from the body, especially immediately following treatment. I was very conscious of drinking enough water at that time as I wanted to flush all chemicals out of my body as quickly as possible. I had to believe this was a good thing to do for my body.

The Lark newsletter of June 2004 shared a survey conducted by the Centers for Disease Control and Prevention. The topic was alternative medicine use. Resouces were those listed on the next page.

Most Popular Complementary and Alternative Health Care Resources

1. Prayer for one's own health
2. Prayer by others for one's own health
3. Natural products (vitamins, minerals, herbs, enzymes)
4. Deep breathing exercises
5. Participation in prayer groups for one's own health
6. Meditation
7. Chiropractic care
8. Yoga
9. Massage
10. Diet-based therapy

*Cast all your anxiety on Him
because He cares for you.*

—1 Peter 5:7

~12~

Dealing with Stress

I am convinced that years of stress contributed to my vulnerability to cancer. The increasing demands in my life put enormous pressure on my mind and body. I had a stressful management job. But I regarded myself as a capable problem-solver, and a manager who possessed enough self-confidence and education to handle almost any situation. Cancer forced me to face my limitations and made me realize that sometimes we are given seemingly impossible tasks.

When stress is long-term, it can affect us physically, emotionally, and spiritually, all impacting our well-being. When we are under stress, worried, or thinking negative thoughts, we are more likely to get sick. Stress has definite physical effects, but it often takes years to notice them. Long-term stress changes the balance of hormones in the body and leads to exhaustion. A suppressed immune system, slower metabolism and slower rate of cell repair result in a variety of problems including minor illnesses, psychological burn-out, and a greater risk of degenerative disease.

If we recognize stress, we need to look for positive things we can do to improve our outlook. When feeling stressed, I ask myself the question, "What difference will this make tomorrow?" It restores my perspective.

Managing stress involves three major elements:
1. Changing the external situation.
2. Changing the way we respond to the situation.
3. Changing the way we perceive or interpret the situation.

Upon hearing the second diagnosis in 2002 I made a major decision about retirement. I left my job within three weeks of hearing the news that the cancer was back. I had not planned to retire for several years. However, I very suddenly knew it was time to go and I did. I could no longer waste time on the concerns of the job. My new job was to rid myself of stress by walking away from my many responsibilities. Retirement required a major restructuring of my life.

Stress cannot be ignored. It must be recognized and treated, or physical difficulties will develop at some point. We can learn and practice stress reduction techniques. We can always seek serenity. We can socialize and stay connected to family and friends. We can think about the good memories, the happy times, and the blessings we have received. We can create a peaceful, easy feeling for ourselves. Stress and worry are a waste of time. Control is an illusion. Let go, let God.

Did you know?

1. Our immune system is strengthened by kindness.
2. An act of kindness will benefit the giver and receiver from a rise in serotonin levels.*
3. An observer of an act of kindness also receives a boost in serotonin levels.

*Serotonin is a neurotransmitter—a chemical that transmits information between nerve cells. It affects how one feels emotionally and physically.

Immune System Boosters

1. Spend more time with family and friends.
2. Volunteer time to favorite causes.
3. Take up a hobby.
4. Attend church services.
5. Get a pet.
6. Exercise with a friend.
7. Eat more fruits and vegetables each day.
8. Get eight hours of sleep each night.
9. Pay attention to emotional health.
10. Laugh more often.

NOTES

*This is a day which the Lord has made;
rejoice and be glad in it.*
—Psalm 118:24

~13~

Focus on Others

Volunteer commitments helped me focus on others rather than dwelling on illness. I realized how much certain causes meant to me. I believe the greatest gift we can give someone is our time. Volunteering is a most fulfilling deed. Researchers have documented that volunteering provides a sense of competence and accomplishment and serves as an antidote to stress and depression. As volunteers we will get back so much more than we give. These are some of the organizations I am committed to help.

American Cancer Society (ACS)
I believe ordinary people can do extraordinary things in the fight against cancer, especially at the local level. I am involved with the annual ACS

Relay for Life fundraiser. My church sponsors a team in this event. ACS is a nationwide non-profit community-based health organization dedicated to eliminating cancer. Its mission is to prevent cancer, save lives, diminish suffering through research, education, advocacy, and service to the public.

March of Dimes
The March of Dimes is another non-profit organization. Its mission is to improve the health of babies by preventing birth defects and infant mortality. It was founded in 1928 when President Roosevelt asked citizens to send a dime to Washington D.C. to help find a cure for polio. The response was overwhelming. My interest in this organization is a result of having survived polio. It was only through the financial generosity of people across this country that the dream of conquering polio became a reality.

Today's March of Dimes has shifted its focus to newborn babies. This organization currently supports research, community services, education, and advocacy programs to eradicate birth defects. In 2003 it launched a five-year campaign to address the increasing rate of premature birth. Its mission is for all babies to be born healthy. I strongly support this cause because of the death of my great-granddaughter, sweet baby Alyssa.

Outreach Literacy Council Program
Another cause I am involved with is literacy. It is one of my passions and offers great rewards to both student and tutor. Tutors are trained to teach English as a second language, reading, and writing skills using the Frank Laubach method, now under the ProLiteracy umbrella. Tutors work one-on-one, teaching everyday living skills as well as English, thus helping students successfully integrate and adapt to their new community. One of the strengths of the program is making new friends and learning about their culture.

The program has expanded my perception of the world. I have worked with six different Hispanic, Hmong, and Chinese ESL students since 1997. All have touched my heart and I am a better person as a result. I am the lucky one in this situation. Volunteering is one of my cures for whatever ails me and is a constant reminder of how blessed I am.

Consider this quote by Albert Pine: "What we do for ourselves dies with us. What we do for others is and remains immortal."

~IV~

To Heal Again

I thank God upon every remembrance of you.
—Philippians 1:3

~14~

Mom, My Hero

When I was diagnosed with cancer, my mind raced back to 1965 when my mother's cancer ordeal began with a radical mastectomy. We are on a different path now than we were thirty-five years ago. Cancer has only been considered a somewhat treatable disease for the past several decades. New opportunities and options have been developed that were unimaginable prior to 1970, when my mother died. Many cancers, such as breast cancer, are curable using today's techniques.

Fighting cancer means facing our own mortality. Mom's mastectomy was followed by brutal chemotherapy with no effective anti-nausea drugs. In 1967 her gallbladder was removed. Within one year she had a hysterectomy, which was again followed by brutal chemotherapy. It was difficult to watch.

Mom had three surgeries plus two rounds of chemotherapy in a five-year period. She was hospitalized and starting the third series of chemo when she passed away. She was like a lamb led to the slaughter. She was so incredibly brave and so very sick from her treatments, which were primitive at that time. The last injection was given directly into her stomach. I don't know how she endured it. Her treatment was experimental and unfortunately, that was all that was available. People like Mom were the real pioneers in cancer treatment. She made it easier for me and for others many years later.

A quick sketch of Mom reveals a wise, strong, courageous woman, personable, and well-liked by everyone who knew her. She was a beautiful person, inside and out. She had grown up during the Depression. She was left a widow with four children at age thirty-four, when my father died of acute leukemia. He was only thirty-five. There were no grief counselors in those days. My family simply accepted its fate and moved on. There was never even a trace of bitterness or depression in Mom that my child's brain could detect.

While looking for the good at every turn, Mom clung to her faith in God and believed that everyone's heart was "in the right place." She never complained. Through trial and tribulation she remained the sweetest thing. My mom was a central force in my life. We were very close. She was crazy about her grandchildren, and living in the same community, we saw each other frequently. She was the role model of everything good. She came as close to being a living saint as any mortal could. I say this because everyone who knew her would agree.

Mom's homespun wisdom keeps coming back to me. "No time like the present" was one of her motivators. Her life philosophy was, "If you can't say anything nice, don't say anything." I recall her expression of, "Where do you go when your back is against the wall?" That is where cancer put her in 1965. She was a woman determined to maintain normalcy for everyone in her family. I remember our disagreement regarding her need to scrub and wax the kitchen floor before entering the hospital the last time. She left everything in apple-pie order. "Be gentle with yourself" would never have occurred to her. Like most women of her generation, she put everyone else's needs first. She did what was expected and kept her problems private.

I miss my mother's wisdom, her goodness, and her grace. I think of her every time I enter a hospital. To this day I truly regret not doing more to help her because I simply didn't know what more to do, other than to be there. Now I understand how important it is just to be there. Mom's courage and strength were my guiding lights. She was a hero to me. My memories of her helped me stay the course. Improvement in medical science made cancer less traumatic for me. Mom "paid it forward." She and other pioneers paved the way for all of us who came after.

What is a hero? The dictionary states it is any person admired for courage. Heroes serve as models to the rest of us, demonstrating exemplary behavior by facing tremendous adversity and adjusting to it. They do not lose hope or give up. We need inspiration and illumination in our lives. Heroes are problem solvers who light the path by providing shining examples for those who follow. They are teachers, and we have much to learn. I was blessed with many heroes who inspired me. My favorite aunt and my fifth-grade teacher had a huge influence on my life. The "Mother Teresas" in my life are the ordinary people doing extraordinary things for others in need.

Many heroes have had outstanding success in life, but often their claim to fame is not based on their talents, but personal victories. When it comes to cancer, Lance Armstrong stands out as a hero. He battled and won victory over testicular cancer. His bicycle ride through the French Alps proved life's suffering can inspire success. What he learned from cancer helped him grow stronger. His advice at the finish line in Paris was, "If you ever get a second chance in life for something, you've got to go all the way." He continues to win and is a constant inspiration to many.

Christopher Reeve qualifies as a hero for me as well. Survival is the most powerful concept in his story. He faced tremendous adversity after a fall from his horse. The resulting paralysis left him immobilized, but he never gave up. He fought incredible odds and became an advocate for every disease victim. His activism was not limited to finding a cure for his own affliction. He fought for medical research across the board. Christopher Reeve's strength and passion caught and held my attention and admiration when I needed courage to face my illness.

Draw near to God and He will draw near to you.
—James 4:8

~15~

Power of Faith

Since I first received a wake-up call from God ten years ago, ideas kept bumping around in my brain about disease and recovery. Is there more to recovery from disease than correct diagnosis and the proper treatment? I think there is. Could people have an intuitive sense of direction for their healing? Yes, they can! Prayer is the key. When we pray we stop trying to control our lives. After all, it's already taken care of for us. Faith is a knowing that God will do what is right for us. Our destiny is in His hands. He is the healer of all ills.

I believe God is the one who hears our prayers. God's help is near if we seek it. Prayer is a divine weapon against all ills, as well as the way to know God. Faith, hope, and love have a strong connection. What we hope for is tied to the kind of faith we have. A lack of hope can kill. An ancient proverb states, "He who has faith has hope, and he who has hope has everything."

Prayer is easier than we think. It is real contact with God. It is sustenance for the soul. There are many kinds of prayer—gratitude, supplication (for ourselves), exhortation (for others), adoration, confession, and forgiveness. Prayer has different meanings for each of us. Prayer gives me a sense of purpose, vision, and meaning for my life. It also provides a feeling of security. It helps me cope with the stress of life by giving me the courage to persevere. It is a tremendous resource of strength I draw from each day.

In addition, prayer has a positive influence on health and well-being. We need the personal connection to God. I turn my problems over to the Lord and let Him lead. I have heard people say, "There is nothing left to do but pray." I say, "Try prayer first." God is listening. God will provide. Only with His help was I able to make it through all of the medical procedures that two episodes of cancer required. Many times I would start with "Help me survive for the next five minutes, the next hour, or the next day." I never could have come this far without His help. Prayer brought me through many stressful situations.

Power of Faith

When first diagnosed I was quite unprepared for the end of life. My interest in prayer peaked then and has never diminished. At that time I tuned into a Christian radio station each day while commuting to work. I heard Bible basics, thanks to a radio signal. It was a great review for me. Was it a coincidence? I don't think so; rather, it was by design. I have always known simple statements like "God loves me," or "God loves everyone." But it was profound, hearing it again—almost like a revelation. I believe we are all creations of God. He loves sinners as much as saints. Prayer is all about God and our loving connection to Him. I pray about everything and pray continuously.

How should we pray? How often to pray? When do we pray? It's all up to us. I set aside a quiet time to approach God each day. It quickly became what I think of as an ongoing dialogue with God. I also go through my day taking a minute for simple prayers, as my thoughts trigger them. I find prayer most helpful when I just open my heart and talk. A simple "Thank you, God" keeps me in touch with the blessings flowing my way each day. Prayer keeps me grounded, helps me maintain my perspective on life, and does wonders for my mood. "Grant me the wisdom to understand" is another frequent prayer of mine.

My thoughts were nonstop and scattered for a long time. I realized I needed to get my inner life in balance. Solitude is a great gift for this purpose. Many times as a child I was told, "Silence is golden." I never appreciated solitude until adulthood. Now I treasure it. It offers a chance to be comfortable alone. Time spent alone leads to awareness of my deepest feelings. I take time to be by myself, to be quiet, to just be. In the past I was always in a hurry. I was distracted by trivial matters. I have learned to slow down. I love Sundays. God gave us the Sabbath as a day of rest.

I believe human beings have a need to believe in something divine. Time and time again I have seen God at work in my life. It is reassuring in hindsight to realize how the pieces of my life fit together. I now look for God's hand in the unexpected things happening in my life. As a result of talking to God, I have the courage to follow my heart and intuition. The message in the Bible is timeless, and I find the word of God has answers for me.

I believe God performs miracles for us all the time—our eyes must be open to see them. Awareness is key. We cannot make complete sense of our lives. This is where faith and trust come in. We don't need to be afraid to ask for a miracle. His ways are not our ways. He will provide the right miracle at the right time. This explains why we don't always recognize a miracle. God knows everything about us, and therefore, He knows which miracle is best. Life is not about what I want, but about what God has planned for me. It never was about me.

Part of my faith is my belief in angels. In the past few years, a great deal of attention has been paid to angels. There are many references to angels in the Bible. In both Hebrew and Greek, the word for angel is "messenger."

Many people are aware of insight and guidance offered at surprising times. I believe that information is from God, delivered to me by angels. I believe some of my friends are angels. We can be open to angels working behind the scenes to carry out God's plans.

Early during chemo treatment in 1996, I was up after a restless night. I thought I might feel better if I accomplished something, so I gathered a laundry basket and headed for the laundromat. I spotted a female in the parking lot. When I reached the door of the building, the same woman held it open for me. I thanked her, started my laundry, and opened my book, placing the bookmark on the table. Shortly thereafter this woman literally loomed over me from behind. She tapped on my bookmark. I looked up at her and she said,

"It's true, you know." I glanced at the bookmark to refresh my memory and turned to respond, but she had vanished. I stood up and looked for her; she wasn't in the building. I returned to my book, looking at the bookmark inscription. It read "God works in mysterious ways." I knew she was a messenger.

In 1999 I was reassigned to an office forty-five miles from my home. It was a longer commute on a dangerous road, and I simply hated the entire scenario. The day I learned the reassignment news at work, I had a conversation with God on the drive home. I outlined all the reasons I thought the job change was not a good idea for me. Finally I surrendered and said, "Okay God, I just don't get it. But if that's where you want me, then that is where I will be."

On my very first day at the new office, my staff presented me with a bumper sticker that read, "Pray for me—I drive Highway 10." I continually searched for a shorter, faster route. I found a back road that left Highway 10 but required crossing busy highways at a sharp curve. One day, reaching the crossway, I stopped, looked both ways, and started forward. I heard a man's voice inside my car state very emphatically, "Look again!" I did, and saw an approaching vehicle that had been hidden in the curve. It most certainly would have broadsided my car on the driver's side. It would have been a disaster for me. I was shaking and praised God the remainder of the drive. I know an angel was in the car with me that day. I never took that route again.

I believe God placed me in that new job, in that particular community, to learn more about courage from my nephew, Dennis, who lived there with his parents. He had been battling cancer since age fourteen. I feel so privileged that I came to know him and witness what a fine adult he came to be. He was a terrific son, brother, grandchild and nephew. He was fun-loving, oh so brave, and courageous. He fought hard for nearly ten years.

He had a gift for those of us he left behind—his testimony that Jesus was there for him on the night he died. His priest arrived that final night and moved to sit near the bed. Dennis told him he could not sit in that particular chair. The priest asked Dennis who was in the room. He answered, "My mom, my dad, Jesus, and you." Jesus was there to take Dennis home. That was a stunning announcement! What a gift he gave to his family and friends.

Six weeks after his death, I visited the cemetery and found grass growing over the grave. I realized that my work there was finished. I had just been reassigned back to my home community. To me that was further proof of how God works in mysterious ways. God, placed me near Dennis for a while to learn from him. Now it was time for me to move on.

    I know there are angels on earth. They have walked beside me all my life. Following the second cancer episode in 2003 I was scheduled to have my port removed. I was on my knees, praying, because I just couldn't go through the procedure alone. The surgeon had questioned me about its removal, but favored leaving it in. He asked what I would do if I ever needed it again. I had responded that I would cross that bridge if I ever came to it. Once I was prepped, the doctor entered the room. His nurse immediately moved to my side and took my hand and held it through the entire procedure. She was an angel to me. I will never forget that act of kindness. I was so thankful God had answered my prayer. I believe I have a guardian angel and that we all do. We can learn to recognize the "coincidences" and miracles in our lives. I think our angels are all around us.

WHAT CANCER CANNOT DO

Cancer is so limited—
It cannot cripple love,
It cannot shatter hope,
It cannot corrode faith,
It cannot destroy peace,
It cannot kill friendship,
It cannot suppress memories,
It cannot silence courage,
It cannot invade the soul,
It cannot steal Eternal Life,
It cannot conquer the Spirit.
 —Anonymous

A friend loves at all times.
—Proverbs 17:17

~16~

I'm Still Me

I am a cancer survivor, but I am still me! I will always be me, and you will always be you. Just like a snowflake or a star, we are each unique creations with gifts and resources which are all on loan to us from God. Our families, friends, and life experiences shape the people we are today. I am indeed the same person who was given the diagnosis of cancer, but deeper and more complex than I was prior to illness.

People and their conditions are not one and the same. I found this to be true when I discovered I had become a faceless, nameless "lymphoma" to others. I didn't like it. As a result I developed great empathy for the less fortunate. I believe instead of labeling people who have physical, mental, or emotional problems, we need to think of how difficult life must be for them. I often think about the everyday activities I take for granted, like walking and talking. A little understanding about impairments goes a long way. We are all less than perfect. People with disabilities are still human beings.

We can learn from and even benefit from talking with those who've had serious illnesses or medical problems. As my seemingly endless treatments went on, I faithfully wrote in my journal. I developed lists of coping skills for surviving cancer. They helped me through my toughest times. My mantra became "Nothing is hopeless" and I repeated it many times each day.

I continually asked, "What am I to learn from this experience?" Finally, the pieces of the puzzle started coming together. The answers were clearer. I have a new awareness of life in general. Life is what we make it. My belief system has expanded. There are no black or white situations, only many shades of gray, and sometimes even mauve or chartreuse. Human beings are very capable of adapting to changing situations. I am a better person as a result of coping with cancer, living life, meeting its challenges, and looking for the best in others and in myself.

Serious illness changed my life, my image of myself, and quite possibly the image others have of me. One person's illness never occurs in a vacuum. It touches many lives. It literally puts one in someone else's hands. We may lose autonomy and power, become dependent on others, and strangers may provide our care. On the day of the first diagnosis I made a giant leap forward into the unknown. The momentum of events took me where there were no rules. I went into treatment not knowing how to handle it. Intellectually and emotionally this was a tremendous challenge, a traumatic time. I couldn't come out of an experience with cancer the same person I was when I first heard the news. It's not possible. But even though I felt my body had betrayed me, leaving me broken and shattered, I found I could recover and go on.

What I needed was hope to go on. I was feeling lost and alone. Cancer got my attention. It temporarily took over my life. How do we find the strength to face each day with a life-threatening disease hanging over our heads? Only later would I understand that real strength comes from within. Faith in God was my strength. Time alone to think and write in my journal helped me sort through many emotions. My life began to change for the better. I learned to put my energy into things I believed in. My life is not the same now, but it's still my life. Am I back to normal? No, but that is only because normal has changed.

The "new me" came to accept that I would be okay with whatever happened next. Now I see each day as an adventure. Life is more than just surviving. It's truly living while we are alive. I believe everything that happens to us has spiritual significance. Things happen for a reason. A person who has had cancer once may be at higher risk for another independent cancer, as well as for a recurrence. The longer we are able to hold cancer at bay, the better our chances for preventing it, and for having a long life. As post-cancer patients, we need to be doubly aware that preventative measures are the best way to avoid cancer. Protecting ourselves from getting cancer again is always in the back of our minds. The post-treatment phase can be a time of anxiety and depression or it can be just the opposite. I try to make it the opposite.

One good day is worth two unknown tomorrows. The gift of wisdom is in accepting that our path has changed—that false illusions and expectations are gone. Acceptance of an imperfect reality is a sign of faith in God. I wanted to believe that something good could come out of my experience with cancer. I'm convinced that God gave me the gift of recovery for a reason. I feel compelled to make good use of my time. The Bible says, "To whom much has been given, of him much is expected." (Luke 12:48) I do believe we are here on earth to help each other, and that life is about letting God use us for his purposes.

What Cancer Taught Me

1. Surrender your life to God.
2. Ignore statistical odds; many people beat them.
3. Reframe your issues to make life easier.
4. Focus on the things that matter most to you.
5. Life is not ordinary. Every day is a mystery.
6. Don't put off anything until tomorrow.
7. Appreciate the others in your life.
8. Just show up and do it.
9. Think about how God has blessed you.
10. Each day is a gift from God.

*The prayer of a righteous man is
powerful and effective.*

—James 5:16

~17~

Gift from God

My faith has been strengthened by illness. It makes sense to take care of our bodies, and our psychological well-being is an important component of our health. However, even if we're conscientious and do all the right things, we may still get sick. A life-threatening diagnosis places us in a whole new world. Remember the question Bernie Siegel asked, "What are the benefits of having this disease?" Now I can answer that question. I found the time to think my own thoughts, to listen to my authentic self, to be truly present in the moment. I no longer put anything off for tomorrow. I moved forward on my faith journey, finding it easier to forgive myself and others. I thank God for every day I am given, and I live life with faith, hope, and love.

Illness taught me some of the truest things in life. We are not here forever. We will all die; no one escapes it. Our time is limited, so it is important to get our affairs in order. Every day I count my blessings. I do each day whatever I can to assure my appreciation carries over to those I love and those who love me. We are what we love, a composite of the many roles we played during our lifetimes, but most of all, we are a work in progress.

Remission brought me to a new phase of life. I recall a cold, sunny day in January of 2003. I had officially retired from my job that month, and had just been given a new lease on life. After leaving my oncologist's office, I walked along the shores of Lake Michigan. Tears were freezing on my face as I thanked God for the gift of remission. God is always with me, closest when I am unsure where the road is taking me. What could I do in return for this gift of life? I prayed for the wisdom to understand what I was to do with this time he was giving me.

The word "remission" is very liberating. It means regaining our sense of normalcy. It is also a challenging phase and can be a difficult time in a cancer patient's life. Some people suffer delayed stress reactions. Many have problems fitting back into their old lives because cancer has changed them. The same skills we learned to fight cancer can help rebuild our lives when in remission. The emotional recovery from cancer can take longer than the physical recovery. Cancer is an experience outside the norm. It is traumatic. As post-cancer patients, we feel vulnerable. We need to watch for signs of stress. Close monitoring of tumor markers, along with other medical testing helps provide a sense of well-being. It is not unusual to spend a year or more rebuilding strength and resiliency. We need to be more vigilant regarding our nutrition, rest, and exercise. Our goal is to reduce our cancer risk. Lifestyle changes offer no guarantees but do increase our chances of a longer life.

When we are seriously ill, the moment of truth has arrived. It's a time to examine what we really want in our lives. Evaluation is a healing process because it opens one to hope and new directions. It is also learning to accept people and situations while concentrating on becoming a better person. I try to remember that change is inevitable, that everything is tenuous at best. In fact, change is the only constant in life.

Illness taught me more about patience than I could ever have imagined. God gave me patience and courage to meet my challenges. I learned I could be scared and still go on. I learned about inner strength and resilience. I learned to recognize and acknowledge each day as a gift from God.

We can fill a new day any way we want. I believe the choice is ours because God gave us choice. Happiness is a choice. When I follow my heart, I can't go wrong. I'm convinced that if we made all decisions from love, we could end pain and suffering in our lives. I try to put my energy into things that are of eternal significance. My relationship with God is precious to me.

I believe the purpose of life is to grow into the best human beings we can be. Our character is developed through trials. There is great wisdom in remaining open to the possibility of growth in any or all circumstances. John Lennon wrote, "Life is what happens to you while you are busy making other plans." And, far earlier than Lennon's era, Leo Tolstoy wrote, "True life is lived when tiny changes occur."

Every day is a growth opportunity. No action is action. This is an important concept. No matter what we do, life will bring us new experiences and problems to solve. I believe God will be walking with us as we journey through them. Serious illness provides an opportunity for faith to deepen and grow.

When first diagnosed with cancer I felt betrayed and mistrustful of my body and of life.

Gift from God

At the end of treatment I felt profound gratitude for my body's ability to withstand treatment and heal again. I had a new appreciation for courage and determination. I am now a person who has had cancer. I refuse to waste my time thinking about cancer. I have more important things to do with my time. I have set my sights on good health and happiness. I practice thankfulness, surround myself with family photos as a reminder of those I love, and I make room for the sacred in my life. I embrace each day, thanking God I am alive and well.

I pray for all people facing cancer. I pray that you, like me, will be blessed with an outpouring of the kind of caring that both humbled and strengthened me. I will be eternally grateful to all who sent me messages of hope and love. As God is in control, all is well with my soul. May God bless you, and always keep you in His light.

Acknowledgements

To my children, Kathy, Steve, and Dave, and all of my family, friends, co-workers, neighbors and medical staff who were there for me during the long journey through cancer both the first and second time. I thank all of you who kept me grounded and hopeful during treatment. I can never properly repay your many kind deeds. Your presence meant the world to me. I couldn't have survived without your encouragement. My eternal gratitude and my wish for each and every one of you is a long and happy life.

BOOK ORDER FORM
(please copy and fill out)

To order your copy or copies of *Faith, Hope, and Cancer: A Survior's Tips* by Carol Westfahl, please provide the following information:

Name: _____

Address: _____

City: _____ State: _____ Zip: _____

Email: _____

Phone: _____

Quantity __ x $13.95: _____

S & H: _____

Subtotal: _____

If ordering from WI, please add 5.5% sales tax to subtotal: _____

Order Total: _____

Shipping & Handling:
$5.00 for 1st book, $1.25 per book thereafter. Unless otherwise requested, books will be sent by USPS media mail.

Method of Payment: ❏ Check ❏ Money Order ❏ Visa ❏ Mastercard

For quantity discounts, please contact the author directly at www.faithhopeandcancer.com

Credit Card Number: _____ Exp. Date: _____

Signature: _____

Please copy this order form and send with payment to:

Faith, Hope, and Cancer
Attn: Carol Westfahl
P.O. Box 1802
Manitowoc, WI 54221-1802

Thank you for your order!